Traditional Chinese Therapeutic Exercises and Techniques

INFANTILE TUINA THERAPY

Written by   Luan Changye
Illustrated by   Shan Yongjin
Translated by   Fang Tingyu, Zhang Kai
and Su Zhihong

FOREIGN LANGUAGES PRESS   BEIJING

First edition   1989

ISBN 0-8351-2150-X   ISBN 7-119-00641-X

Copyright 1989 by Foreign Languages Press, Beijing, China

Published by Foreign Languages Press
24 Baiwanzhuang Road, Beijing, China

Printed by Foreign Languages Printing House
19 West Chegongzhuang Road, Beijing, China

Distributed by China International Book Trading Corporation
(Guoji Shudian), P.O. Box 399, Beijing, China

Printed in the People's Republic of China

About the Author

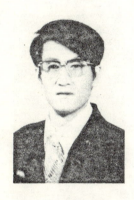

Luan Changye, a tuina specialist of the traditional Chinese Medicine Section of Weihai Sanatorium, Shandong Province, was born in Gaixian County, Liaoning Province, in 1937. At sixteen he began studying tuina therapy and acknowledges more than ten tuina specialists in China as his masters. During thirty-some years of tuina research and clinical experience he has contributed twenty-four special articles to medical magazines in China and published four monographs and a set of tuina illustrations.

Drawing on his own and others' clinical experience and research, he has developed six commonly used manipulations and a unique school of tuina. A renowned tuina specialist in China, he is Vice President of the Shandong Tuina Society, President of the Yantai Tuina Society and General Secretary of the Weihai Traditional Chinese Medicine Society.

Preface

Tuina, also known as massage, is an important component of traditional Chinese recovery therapy in which diseases are cured by the operator's manipulations on the patient's body to stimulate the meridians, collaterals and points. The earliest record of tuina treatment in China was seen in *The Yellow Emperor's Internal Classic*, a medical treatise published in the fifth century B.C. "Blood, Qi, and Mental-Physical Conditions" is a chapter relating to tuina treatment of diseases. It points out, "When a person is in frequent shock and the passages of the meridians and collaterals are blocked, disease attacks him mostly in the form of numbness, and it should be treated by massage." This indicates that tuina therapy is able to promote the circulation of qi and blood, remove the obstruction of the meridians and collaterals, and benefit joint movement. The biophysical and biochemical changes of the muscles resulting from massage are evident. These biological changes invigorate lymphatic flow, facilitate blood circulation, and strengthen the metabolism, thus reducing swelling, preventing hemorrhage and old bleeding (also called "eliminating the stale and the stagnant" in the *Internal Classic*), tonifying the tendons and bones, strengthening the contraction of the ligaments, and playing a bilateral function in sedating the nerves and inhibiting analgesia. All these facts have proved that tuina therapy is able to relieve organic diseases and to eliminate functional disturbance. This therapy is simple, economical and free from side-effects, sparing not only infants from the bitterness of medication and the pain of injections, but also their parents from worry. Infants cooperate with and easily accept this therapy because the manipulations produce comfortable sensations on their body surfaces.

I have engaged in clinical and theoretical research on traditional Chinese recovery for more than forty years. I was pleased to read the new book *Infantile Tuina Therapy* written by Dr. Luan Changye and was deeply impressed by his concern for the health of the people. The theories of the book are well grounded, the methods of treatment numerous and the results effective. Dr. Luan Changye has been working in tuina for thirty years. His clinical experience is abundant and his academic achievement great. He has written *Massage Therapy*, *Tuina Therapy* and *The Illustrated Infantile Tuina Therapy*. His *Hanging Charts of Tuina Therapy* is the first coloured edition for adults in China, and fills a gap in the field of tuina science in China. He has made a definite contribution to the development of traditional Chinese recovery. I am pleased to have had this chance to preface this book. I am confident that readers will gradually experience the true essence of this book and will find it inspiring and instructive. I heartily recommend this book in China and abroad, and I trust that it will benefit infants all over the globe.

Professor Hu Bin

*Member of the Specialist Information
Committee, China Academy of
Traditional Chinese Medicine
December 3, 1985*

Contents

I. Background and Introduction to Infantile
   Tuina Therapy   1
1. A Short History of Infantile Tuina Therapy   1
2. Characteristics of Infantile Tuina Therapy   3
3. How Tuina Therapy Works   5
4. Physiological and Pathological Features of
   Infants   9

II. Diagnosis of Infantile Patients   11
1. Four Diagnostic Methods   12
2. Analysis and Differentiation of Pathological
   Conditions in Accordance with the Eight
   Principal Syndromes   25

III. Commonly Used Manipulations in Infantile
   Tuina Therapy   26

IV. Points Frequently Used in Infantile
   Tuina Therapy   36
1. Points on the Head and Face   36
2. Points on the Back   46
3. Points in the Thoracic and Costal Regions   52

4. Points in the Medial Aspect of the Upper
   Limbs and Palm 59
5. Points Along the Lateral Aspect of the Upper
   Limbs and the Dorsum of the Palm 76
6. Points of the Lower Limbs 85

V. Indications of the Commonly Used Points and
   Prescriptions for Common Infantile Diseases ... 91

VI. Precautions 105
1. Mediums to Be Used 105
2. Reinforcing-Reducing Method and
   Reinforcing-Reducing Intensity 105
3. Position 106
4. Tuina Sequence 106
5. The Principle of Treatment and Prescriptions .. 107

VII. Classification Table for the Commonly Used
     Tuina Points 109

I. Background and Introduction to Infantile Tuina Therapy

Tuina therapy, a traditional Chinese treatment thousands of years old, is a kind of remedial massage. Infantile tuina therapy, an adaptation of the therapy for adults, is commonly regarded as the best form of treatment for babies because it has a wide range of indications, is simple, safe, painless and inexpensive, and because it produces no side effects and requires a shorter course of treatment.

1. A Short History of Infantile Tuina Therapy

Although there were no monographical writings on infantile tuina therapy prior to the Ming Dynasty (1368-1644), ancient medical literature suggests that the treatment was being used in far earlier times. One of the first systematic descriptions of tuina therapy for infants was provided by Mr. Chen in his *Infantile Remedial Massage*, which was included in Yang Jizhou's *Compendium of Acupuncture and Moxibustion* of 1601. Chen's work discusses the manipulations, regions for treatment and diagnosis, with particular attention given to the examination of the finger venules of infants. In 1604, Gong Yunlin offered a more systematic description of the therapy based on his own experience in his *Guide to Infantile Tuina Therapy*. This illustrated work, which describes infantile diseases in rhymed songs and discusses diagnosis, manipulations and points, laid a reliable foundation for the development and popularity of infantile tuina therapy.

In 1676, the tuina specialist Xiong Yunying compiled and published the three-volume *A General Description of Infantile Tuina Therapy*. The first volume treats the principles of tuina therapy and diagnostic methods for infantile diseases with about twenty illustrations of the manipulations. The second volume describes clinical treatment of common infantile diseases. This book was popular because it combined theory with practice. In his five-volume *Essentials of tuina Therapy*, Luo Rulong, a paediatrician and infantile tuina specialist, describes in detail medical examination, tuina points, and the manipulations used for various infantile conditions. In 1776, Qian Ruming revised and republished the clinically useful *Secrets of Infantile Tuina Therapy* by Zhou Yufan of the Ming Dynasty. The first volume of this work discusses diagnosis and manipulations and the second deals with case analysis and clinical therapy with illustrations.

The proliferation of fundamental works on infantile tuina therapy during the Ming and Qing dynasties gave rise to the notion that the therapy began then. This popular form of treatment flourished during those times, and even though it suffered political repression during the Qing (1644-1911), especially from the mid-1800s on, people used it secretly, and infantile tuina therapy advanced further than did the tuina therapy for adults.

In the 1950s, bigger hospitals in China recruited distinguished veteran practitioners of traditional Chinese medicine and restored the practice of the influential traditional medical disciplines. Tuina therapy made unprecedented advances, and clinics and departments of tuina therapy sprang up like mushrooms. In the tumultuous years of the "cultural revolution," however, many tuina practitioners were forced to leave the field, and research on and practice of the therapy came to a standstill. Recent years have seen a revival of tuina therapy. The first tuina therapy symposium was held in Shanghai in 1979, and since then tuina research societies and remedial massage associations have been established one after another in some provinces and municipalities. With these signs that tuina therapy is regaining its former popularity, the future of the field looks promising indeed.

2. Characteristics of Infantile Tuina Therapy

Infantile tuina therapy is particularly effective for conditions such as inability to suck milk, regurgitation of milk, morbid night crying, infantile malnutrition, thrush, numb tongue, acute and chronic infantile convulsions, vomiting, diarrhoea, fever, cold, whooping cough, conjunctivitis, bed-wetting, prolapsed rectum, constipation, infantile muscular wryneck, sequela of polio, and intestinal obstruction due to ascariosis. There are no contraindications to the therapy except severe dermatopathy in the area for manipulation and trauma.

Because the therapy involves manipulations on the surface of the body that produce physiological reactions that restore normal bodily functions and strengthen resistance to pathogenic factors, in effect a kind of passive motorpathy, there are no side effects with proper diagnosis and treatment. Tuina therapy requires no special medication or equipment except adjuvants like talcum, liquid paraffin and a mixture of glycerin and alcohol, and patients can be treated anywhere without being subjected to medications or other medical trauma. For example, whereas Western medicine often advises fasting in the treatment of infantile dyspepsia, tuina therapy produces good results without subjecting the rapidly developing infant to such an unwise practice.

It has been proven that the younger the baby, the shorter the course of tuina treatment. Generally, one to three treatments of fifteen to twenty minutes are sufficient. Instant results can be seen in the treatment of the common cold, cough, regurgitation of milk, morbid night crying, diarrhoea, constipation, retention of urine and intestinal obstruction due to ascariosis. Infantile tuina therapy is also cheaper than other forms of treatment. A cost comparison between tuina therapy and medication for infantile diarrhoea in a Shanghai hospital shows that tuina therapy required only 3.5 treatments costing ¥ 1.40 whereas medication required 8 treatments costing ¥ 12.80. Tuina therapy is cheaper than medication even if more tuina treatments are required or less medication is used.

3. How Tuina Therapy Works

Traditional Chinese medicine holds that the human body is an organic whole, each part of the body being interrelated through the meridians by taking the five *zang* (heart, liver, spleen, lungs and kidneys) and six *fu* (stomach, gallbladder, the three visceral cavities housing the internal organs, bladder, and large and small intestines) organs as the centre. As early as two thousand years ago, the ancients considered the meridian system a network connecting the organs and structures. Physiologically, the system's action is to transport blood and *qi*, or vital energy, maintain the equilibrium of *yin* and *yang*, and defend the body from the invasion of pathogenic factors; pathologically, it is a passage through which pathogenic factors travel.

Normal functioning of the body depends on the dynamic balance of yin and yang, without which the constructive energy, defensive energy, qi and blood cannot circulate smoothly and the skin, flesh, tendons, and five zang and six fu organs cannot be amply nourished through the work of the meridians. The meridians are spread all over the body and when a person is alive they naturally perform their functions. When there is disturbance in the meridian system disease occurs. In the chapter Treatise of Pathogenic Factors of *Miraculous Pivot*,* (*Lin Shu*), it says, "when the lungs and heart are diseased, the pathogenic factors are located in the elbows; pathogenic factors settled in the hypocondriac regions account for a diseased liver;

---

*Miraculous Pivot is the first volume of *Canon of Acupuncture*.

a troubled spleen is manifested by pathogenic factors in the thigh; pathogenic factors behind the knees indicate troubled kidneys." The chapter Treatise of Pains of *Plain Questions** (*Su Wen*) states, "cold located in the Back-Shu points induces pain due to a deficiency in the circulatory system. When pressure is applied to the part, heat is produced and the pain disappears." The above shows that one, when a given organ is in disorder, the pathogenic factors may move to the site of its related meridians where abundant qi is concentrated, causing impeded circulation of its qi and affecting the normal function of the organ; two, when the pathogenic factors invade the meridian pertaining to a particular organ, pathological changes of the organ occur; and three, the part affected by the pathogenic factors is considered the treatment region of the first alternative, for the therapy may regulate the circulation of blood and qi, promote normal functioning of the whole body based on the principle that "obstruction of blood and qi gives rise to pain."

The doctrine of meridians, the guiding principle in acupuncture and tuina therapy, is one of the important components of traditional Chinese medicine. The meridian system makes up a network connecting all the internal organs and tissues and reaching every part of the body. In addition, meridians are the passages in which blood and qi travel, maintaining normal functioning of the body. Blood and qi are considered the essential substances that keep a man alive. The organs and structures of the body are nourished by blood and

---

*Plain Questions is the second volume of *Canon of Acupuncture*.

qi that travel in the meridians. It is the meridian system and its regulatory function that make the body as an organic whole work properly.

Each zang or fu organ has its related meridian, with each having its own course. From the condition of the meridians one can tell the function of their related internal organs. This is the theoretical basis of tuina therapy. The Du Meridian among the eight extra meridians controlling all the yang meridians and regulating their qi is known as the "reservoir of yang meridians," while the Ren Meridian ruling all the yin meridians and regulating their qi is called the "reservoir of yin meridians." The Yangwei and Yinwei meridians connect with the six yin and six yang meridians and help to maintain the equilibrium of the qi in the yin and yang meridians. The establishment of the meridian doctrine is based on the understanding of physiological activities, abnormal manifestations in the course of a disease and the effectiveness of treatment. Tuina therapy is also guided by this doctrine. Different manipulations are applied to a selected part of the body in accordance with various conditions, with the assistance of the conducting capability of the meridians to induce the body resistance, promote the circulation of blood and qi and restore the balance of yin and yang, and finally cure the disease.

In recent years new scientific techniques employed in the medical field have played a positive role in the development of tuina therapy, bringing it to a new level. Two experiments have been done in healthy males at the age of twenty by Professor Lu Yunming, Biology Teaching Section of the Affiliated Hospital,

Qingdao Medical College, Shandong Province, with the assistance of the Tuina Therapy Department of the hospital.

1) Gastric peristalsis was observed before and after tuina therapy

Tuina manipulations were applied to the points strengthening the function of the spleen for ten minutes. The gastric peristalsis was as follows: (~~~~~~), ~~~~~~ . Ten minutes later, counterclockwise manipulation was performed on the Neibagua Point. The gastric peristalsis was recorded like this ~~~~~~ . When the gastric peristalsis returned to normal, the same manipulation was applied for another ten minutes. The gastric peristalsis was ~~~~~~ . The above suggests manipulations on the points strengthening the gastric peristalsis and on the Neibagua Point change the patterns of gastric peristalsis.

2) Observation of the digestion of gastric protein

Three test-tubes were filled with the same amount of gastric juice. The first gastric juice was from a person who had not received tuina therapy, the second was from a person who had received tuina manipulations on the points strengthening the spleen for ten minutes, and the third was from a person who had received the above treatment and manipulations on the Neibagua Point for ten minutes. Then pieces of gastric protein of the same size were placed in the tubes, which were put in an incubator for fourteen hours. It was found that the protein in the last tube had decomposed and there was no change in the protein in the first tube. Other experiments also showed that increased gastric digestion was seen after manipulations on the points to reinforce the spleen, and by far more increased gastric digestion was found when manipulations had been applied to the points strengthening the spleen and to the Neibagua Point.

The experiments prove that tuina therapy may motivate the conveying of the meridians and cure diseases. The manipulation on the hand points of infants to treat diarrhoea and other disorders is based on the above-mentioned mechanism.

4. Physiological and Pathological Features of Infants

As the physiological and pathological features of infants differ from those of adults, different manipulations are employed. An infant begins to adapt to his environment shortly after birth. He has a delicate constitution and his organs lack abundant qi, blood, and organ essense. He is not strong enough to fend off the invasion of pathogenic factors. During this period improper nursing tends to lead to the invasion of pathogenic factors and illness. Infants often have a red complexion, big head and short limbs. The fontanel spot is concave in the incompletely ossified skull. The infant likes to sleep and, except for milk feeding, sleeps nearly all day long. The pulse is quick and changeable. A healthy infant must cry several times a day to exercise its lungs, stomach and intestines for normal digestion. Teeth began to grow six months after birth. Now and then the body temperature rises, along with loss of appetite, vomiting, diarrhoea, fright and such, which are not considered the trauma of disease. The signs disappear by themselves in a few days and treatment is unnecessary.

Inadequate resistance and adaptability of infants to the environment due to a delicate constitution and insufficient blood and qi give rise to susceptibility to six pathogenic factors (wind, cold, summer-heat, damp, dryness and fire) or harm by improper feeding. Ear-piercing noise or sudden fright may lead to convulsions. Apart from this, infantile development is impeded by innate insufficiency or post natal malnutrition. As a result, there may appear delayed closure of the fontanels, retarded standing, walking, hair-growth, tooth eruption and speech, softness of the head, neck, limbs, muscles and mouth, and the baby may tend to suffer measles, skin sores, convulsions, infantile malnutrition, thrush, mumps, whooping cough, etc. The conditions are changeable and worse than those of adults. For example, infantile diarrhoea easily leads to exhaustion of body fluid, or even death by acidosis when not properly treated. Exogenous affection may cause asthma, cough, pneumonia or bronchitis. Some infants often have high fevers as soon as they fall ill, although they are as active as the healthy, and then convulsions follow. With proper diagnosis and treatment, sick infants generally recover more easily than adults because of their vigorous physiological functions and lack of emotional interference.

II. Diagnosis of Infantile Patients

Diagnosis is a doctor's determination of the nature of a disease based on symptoms and signs. Correct diagnosis is the preconditions of proper treatment or otherwise the latter must fail.

Diagnostic methods used in traditional Chinese medicine consist of inspection, auscultation and olfaction, interrogation and pulse feeling, guided by the eight principal syndromes; through them the advance, change and prognosis of a disease can be correctly determined. Among the four diagnostic methods, priority is given to inspection, which is especially important in the treatment of infants because they cannot speak, or, if they can, they still cannot articulate clearly the whole story of the case. Pulse feeling for infants is not so useful since it is quite difficult to distinguish their *cun*, *guan* and *chi* pulses in so small an area. Although the three pulses can be felt with one finger, three fingers are always more precise. A correct diagnosis derives first from inspection, interrogation, and then palpation of the abdomen and examination of the superficial veins of the finger. If possible, routine tests or modern medical approaches are employed to make right diagnosis.

1. Four Diagnostic Methods

1) Inspection

The doctor observes the patient's outward manifestation of vitality, complexion and conditions of configuration, tongue, extreta and secretions to infer the favourable or unfavourable trend of the disease.

Observation of the patient's outward manifestation of vitality It is of great significance in detecting the favourable or unfavourable prognosis of a disease since vitality suggests the ability to stay alive. In *Plain Questions*, it states, "one who is full of vitality lives on vigorously while one who loses vitality is apt to die." Vitality is the lifeline both for adults and infants. Full vitality is manifested by bright eyes, a loud and clear voice, a well-developed body, and normal breath, urination and bowel movements, while loss of vitality is indicated by dull eyes, a haggard look, abnormal breath, constant diarrhoea, and weight loss, which show a severe, critical conditions. The nature of a disease, whether it is of cold, heat, excess or deficiency, and the prognosis can be predicted on the basis of drowsiness, excitement, and inactivity. Peaceful breath and sonorous breath can indicate diseases of cold, heat, excess, deficiency, or abundant cold or heat.

Inspection of the complexion Five colours—blue, red, yellow, white, dark—of the complexion conveyed from the inside to the outside through meridians indicate pathological changes taking place in the corresponding internal organs. The Chinese ancestors held that each colour corresponds to an internal organ, e.g.

blue to the liver, red to the heart, yellow to the spleen, white to the lungs, and dark to the kidneys. In terms of symptoms, a blue face is associated with convulsions, a flushed face, with excessive heat, a yellow face, an impaired spleen or indigestion, a white face, deficiency and cold, and a dark face, severe pain. Blue and dark discolouration on the lips is a critical sign, showing a divorce of yin and yang.

Inspection of the eyes The outward manifestation of the liver is eyes, which are supported by the essence of the five zang organs. From the expression of the eyes, one can see the exogenous affection of cold and wind, indigestion and disorders of the zang-fu organs. Pink eyes with gum suggest excessive heat in the liver; eyes brimming with tears and red eyelids, signs of measles; staring eyes and nebulae, a heat syndrome or infantile malnutrition; dramatically sunk eyesockets, a sign of exhaustion of liver function; sudden blindness, exhaustion of yin and blood; corediastasis, lowered function of the stomach and spleen; and staring eyes with fixed pupils, exhaustion of liver function. In prolonged illness of diseases difficult to cure, dull, yellowish or small pupils may be seen.

Inspection of the nose The outward manifestation of the spleen is the nose. A red, dry nose indicates a heat syndrome and a runny nose, exogenous affection. Thick nasal discharge or dry nostrils means heat in the lung meridian. Flaring the nostrils with more inhalation than exhalation is seen in cases difficult to cure. Flaring of nostrils in a prolonged disease accompanied by shortness of breath and profuse sweating is a sign of exhaustion of the lung.

Inspection of the tongue The outward manifestation of the heart is the tongue, in which internal heat or cold is seen. Check whether the tongue is coated or not. A yellow, white, black or red tongue reflects a condition of cold, heat, deficiency or excess respectively and the seriousness of the case.

A dry and yellow tongue coating indicates abundant internal heat, while a red, hard and cracked tongue means upward invasion of toxic heat. A grey and thin coating is a sign of light pathogenic factors, while a thick, black coating reflects strong pathogenic factors. A baby playing with its tongue suggests internal heat. A chronically ill baby playing with its yellow tongue with white coating means invasion of the stomach by pathogenic factors. A white bordered tongue with a dry coating and black centre proposes a critical conditions.

Inspection of the ears The outward manifestation of the kidney is the ear, where the Shaoyang Meridian passes through. Red ears are a sign of abundant vital energy in the kidney. In this case the patient tends to recover easily. When the ear is red and feels hot, it indicates exogenous affection of cold and wind. Endogenous wind in the liver and fever causes blue veins standing out in the ear. Disorders of the Gallbladder Meridian are shown by sudden ear pain, swollen ears or deafness.

Inspection of lips and mouth The outward manifestation of the spleen is the lips. Dark red lips reveal accumulated heat in the heart and spleen; pale lips, deficiency in the spleen and insufficient blood; and bluish lips and mouth, excess in the liver and deficiency in the spleen. Measures must be taken to prevent convulsions. Since the spleen and the stomach are interiorly-exteriorly related, red lips and vomiting show heat in the stomach, whereas pale lips and vomiting mean deficiency in the stomach. Lips neither red nor pale indicate indigestion and an impaired stomach. Lips failing to cover the teeth is a sign of exhaustion of the spleen. Saliva running along the corners of the mouth implies cold in the spleen and cracked lips mean internal heat. Red swollen lips and mouth are signs of abundant heat, and dark red lips indicate a critical condition. Coarse quick breathing means invasion of excessive pathogenic factors, while faint slow breathing indicates impaired genuine energy. A protrusive mouth, exhalation only, or black lips indicate incurable conditions.

Inspection of the feet and hands It is important to examine the feet and hands of an infantile patient. Bluish fingernails denote cardiac pain, and black nails, exhaustion of the liver. Convulsions are reflected by spasms of the hands and feet and a rigid spine.

Inspection of the superficial veins of the index finger Qian Chongyang, a paediatrician of the Song Dynasty (960-1279) named the first, second and third medial parts of the index finger Wind Pass (the proximal segment), Vital Energy Pass (the middle segment) and Life Pass (the distal segment). This is a special diagnostic method for babies under three. The line that runs from the part of the hand between the thumb and the index finger straight along the medial part to the tip is known as the superficial vein (see Fig.1). Yellow and red veins faintly visible are considered normal. When a baby falls ill, the veins vary in shape and

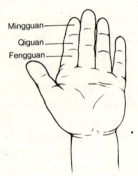

Fig.1 The three passes of the superficial veins of the index finger

colour, which, are valuable in diagnosis. The finger to be inspected should be cleaned with ethyl alcohol and exposed to sunlight. With his thumb, the doctor pushes the medial parts of the index finger upward from the second segment to the first to allow the veins to show.

Vein picture	*Syndrome*
Veins easy to see	Exterior
Veins difficult to see	Interior
Bright red veins easy to see	Exogenous affection
Light red veins	Cold
Purplish veins	Internal heat
Bluish veins	Fright
Black veins	Blood affection

The condition of the disease can be judged by the presence of veins.

Vein presence	Seriousness of diseases
In the first part	Mild
In the second part	Advanced from exterior to interior
In all three parts	Critical

2) Auscultation and olfaction

The voice, sound and odour of a patient are clues to his general condition.

Early Chinese held that sounds and voices are related to the morbid state of the internal organs. A sick baby must have a change in his voice and sound, according to which the doctor can tell the nature of the disease—exterior, interior, cold, heat, deficiency or excess.

Differentiation of exogenous affection and internal injury

Voice and sound	Syndrome
Muffled voice (strong first, feeble later)	Serious exogenous affection
Muffled voice (feeble first, strong later)	Internal injury

Differentiation of cold, heat, deficiency and excess

Syndrome	Disease nature
Fever	Excess
Untalkative cold	Deficiency
Crying with profuse tears	Deficiency
Muffled voice, sneezing	Exogenous excess
Feeble voice, shortness of breath	Deficiency of genuine vital energy

Differentiation of syndromes of the five zang organs

Syndrome	Diseased part
Shortness of breath, asthma	Lung
Shouting, scolding	Liver
Trembling sound	Spleen
Feeble voice	Kidney
Giggling, flat speech	Heart

Differentiation of pains

Syndrome	Pain location
Frowning and groaning	Headache
Loud groaning and touching the chest	Stomachache
Groaning, shaking head, touching the cheeks	Toothache
Groaning and failing to stand	Low back pain

Differentiation of odour

Odour	Disorder
Hot foul breath	Accumulated heat in the stomach
Acid foul breath	Oral sores
Stinking smell	Sinusitis
Acid foul smell of feces	Accumulated heat in the interior
Rotten fish smell	Accumulated cold in the interior
Foul brown urine	Accumulated heat in the bladder
Foul clear urine	Accumulated cold in the bladder

3) Interrogation

Pathological changes before and after the onset of disease

Symptoms after onset	Disorder
Headache, aversion to cold, fever	Exterior
Abdominal pain, diarrhoea, cold sensation in limbs	Interior

Pathological changes	Nature of pathogenic factors or diseases
Restlessness during the day, quiet during the night	Yang
Restlessness during the night, quiet during the day	Yin
Quiet behaviour	Deficiency of vital energy

Restlessness	Strong pathogenic factors
Shortness of breath first, distention second	Lung disorder
Distention first, shortness of breath second	Spleen disorder

Chill and fever

Symptoms	Disorder
Fever, chills, absence of sweating, aversion to wind or spontaneous sweating	Exogenous affection of wind, cold
Fever, sweating, thirst, constipation, brown urine	Abundant internal heat
Persistently feverish sensation of the body and palms	Deficiency of yin due to internal injury
Feeble limbs, grey complexion, pale lips, spontaneous sweating, slight aversion to cold	Deficiency of yang
Preference for cold	Heat syndrome
Preference for heat, chill	Cold syndrome

Sweating

Symptoms	Disorder
Fever, chill, absence of sweating	Exterior, excess
Fever, chill, sweating	Exterior, deficiency
Absence of chill after sweating, fever	Interior

Lassitude, sweating on exertion	Deficiency of yang
Sweating, chill	Exterior
Sweating, absence of chill, aversion to heat	Interior
Dripping with perspiration	Incurable case

Feces and urine

Condition	Syndrome
Loose stool, diarrhoea	Deficiency
Sticky, foul feces	Heat
Watery foul feces	Cold
Constipation with pulse indicating abundant heat	Stasis of yang
Constipation with pulse indicating abundant cold	Stasis of cold
Watery diarrhoea with foul mucoid stools, burning sensation of the anus, pulse indicating abundant heat	Diarrhoea due to heat
Brown urine	Heat
Light coloured urine	Cold
Diarrhoea, brown, scanty urine	Damp and heat
Frequency of urination, bed-wetting	Deficiency of vital energy
Light coloured urine in a baby with a febrile disease	Condition improving

Diet

Normal diet taken means an unimpaired stomach.

Indigestion is manifested by dyspepsia, constipation and eructation.

Symptoms	Disorders
Hunger, no appetite, distress in the stomach	Stomach obstruction by phlegm and fire
More food intake, yet hunger, weight loss	Flamming of stomach fire
Good appetite, abdominal distension	Strong function of the stomach, weak function of the spleen
Abdominal distension after food intake	Stagnation of vital energy and indigestion
Stomachache, abdominal pain relieved after food	Deficiency
Stomachache, abdominal pain, severe after food intake	Excess
Preference for hot diet	Cold in the stomach and intestines
Preference for cold diet	Heat in the stomach and intestines

Thirst

Manifestations	Syndromes
Mad thirst, preference for drinking cold fluids	Interior heat
Preference for profuse drinking	Interior invasion of pathogenic factors of yang
Thirst without desire to drink	Loss of genuine yin

Furthermore, it is important to ask whether the patient has had measles, acute infectious diseases or a smallpox vaccination.

4) Pulse feeling and palpation

We know it is difficult to take pulse in babies. But if extremely necessary, four pulse conditions listed in *A Complete Book of Paediatrics* by Chen Fuzheng of the Qing Dynasty, are introduced below.

Pulse Condition A superficial pulse is felt by light touch. Forceful beating indicates an excess syndrome, while forceless beating reveals a deficiency syndrome, usually seen in exogenous affection of wind and cold.

A deep pulse can be felt while pressing hard, and indicates an interior affection. Forceful beating suggests an interior excess syndrome, and forceless beating, an exterior deficiency syndrome, usually seen in indigestion and stagnation of vital energy.

A slow pulse, which has fewer than 5 to 6 beats to one cycle of respiration, indicates a cold syndrome. Slow but forceful beating implies obstruction and an excess syndrome, and slow and forceless beating, a cold or deficiency syndrome.

A rapid pulse that has more than eight beats to one cycle of respiration, shows a heat syndrome. Forceful beating suggests a heat syndrome of excess, while forceless beating indicates a heat syndrome of deficiency. A superficial and rapid pulse is a sign of an exterior heat syndrome, and a deep and rapid pulse, an interior heat syndrome.

Palpation Palpate the skin lightly to see the condition of dryness or perspiration.

Hard pressure can help determine the degree of

swelling. If the skin returns to normal immediately after pressure and something like water seems surrounded in it, edema is present. If the skin does not return to normal after pressure and it feels thick without change of colour, it is called puffy. If the affected part is soft and hot, pus is present. If the part is hard, pus is not present. Light pressure causing pain indicates pus just below the skin. Hard pressure causing pain means deeper pus. If the skin does not return to normal after pressure, pus is not present, and vice versa.

Palpation of the abdomen In *Treatise on Febrile Diseases* by Zhang Zhongjing of the Han Dynasty (206 B.C.-220), it states, "The five zang and six fu organs are enclosed in the chest and abdomen, where vital energy and blood originate. The condition of the zang-fu organs is predicted by palpation." This approach is highly valued by both modern and traditional medicine in the diagnosis of diseases of the internal organs. Syndromes can be seen in advance based on the pathological changes in the abdomen. If the changes are consistent with the complaints of the patient, proper treatment can be decided upon.

Differentiation of the syndromes

Manifestations	*Syndromes*
Soft abdomen, preference for pressure	Deficiency, cold
Hard abdomen, aggravated by pressure	Excess, heat
Sharp pain, hard abdomen	Excess

Preference for warmth	Cold
Preference for cold	Heat
Distended abdomen, shallow sensation on pressure	Distension due to gas
Flowing of liquid in the abdomen	Accumulation of liquid

2. Analysis and Differentiation of Pathological Conditions in Accordance with the Eight Principal Syndromes

The eight principal syndromes, yin, yang, exterior, interior, heat, cold, deficiency and excess, are the most important distinctions in the differentiation of cases. In terms of category, location and nature of diseases there are only yin and yang, exterior and interior, cold and heat respectively. A case caused by strong pathogenic factors is known as an excess syndrome, while a case caused by lowered body resistance is called a deficiency syndrome. Any disease can be grouped under the eight principal syndromes before an appropriate treatment is decided upon.

III. Commonly Used Manipulations in Infantile Tuina Therapy

Skilful operations have a direct effect on the therapeutic result, so the operator must not only be good at selecting points, but also highly skilled at executing the manipulations to achieve the desired goal.

China has many different schools of tuina therapy and more than a hundred of manipulations, among which only several are adaptable to infants, because infantile disorders are relatively simple and their physiological and pathological features are different from those in adults. The commonly used manipulations are pushing, pulling, pressing, rubbing, rotatory kneading, pinching, kneading, curve pushing, lifting, beating, and shaking.

Appropriate force and frequency are very important in infantile tuina therapy. The best operation is a light-yet-straight or hard-yet-smooth touch, combining hardness with softness. Beginners should first learn to operate in a brisk rhythm, and then operate forcefully with persistance.

Infantile tuina therapy is suitable for babies under five. The younger the patient, the better the results. Some of the adult tuina manipulations may be supplemented for children over five to strengthen the cura-

tive effects.
1) Pushing manoeuvres
Linear pushing The operator holds the patient's wrist or fingers with his left hand and pushes the muscles forcefully forward and backward (see Fig.2) with the pad of the right thumb, index or middle finger.

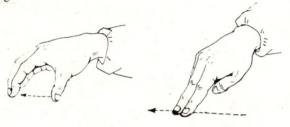

Fig.2 Linear pushing with the thumb and the index finger

The operation should be done linearly so as to avoid other meridians involved. When pushing, use some cream to protect the skin.

Separate pushing The operator pushes the point with his two thumb pads (see Fig.3). This is usually applied to the Kangong, Zanzhu, Xinmen and abdomen points.

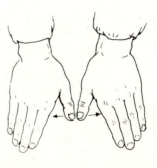

Fig.3 Separate pushing

Rotatory pushing It is

usually applied to the Spleen Meridian by holding the wrist and the thumb of the patient. The operator pushes clockwise with his right thumb pad (see Fig.4).

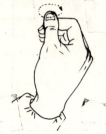

Fig.4   Rotatory pushing

Pushing from the fingertip downward is called the reinforcing method or the reducing method. Upward and downward pushing is known as the clearing method.

2) Pulling manoeuvres

It is done by lifting and squeezing or rapidly releasing the affected muscles, and is usually applied to the Fengchi, Jianjing, Hegu points and both sides of abdomen (see Fig.5).

3) Pressing manoeuvre

The operator's thumb or middle finger presses the selected points with a given force. This is followed by rotatory kneading (see Fig.6). The extent of pressure

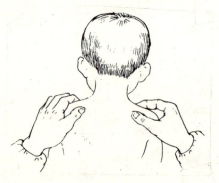

Fig.5   Pulling Jianjing

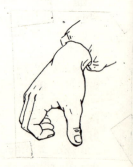

Fig.6   Pressing manoeuvre

must be consistent with the condition, and alternates between light and hard throughout the manoeuvre.

4) Rubbing manoeuvre

It is done with repeated rubbing of the affected part by the operator's index, middle and ring fingers or palm. For rubbing with the finger and palm (see Fig.7),

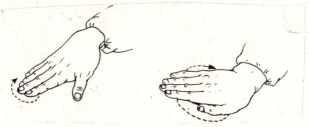

Fig.7 Rubbing with the finger and palm

ascaris and intestinal obstruction respond quickly to rotatory rubbing. The operator rubs the abdomen clockwise over the colon ascendens, transverse colon and colon descendens until the abdomen becomes soft (see Fig.8).

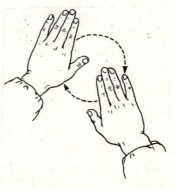

Fig.8 Rotatory rubbing

5) Rotatory kneading manoeuvres

Finger rotatory kneading The operator kneads a given part or point of a patient with his index and middle fingers or index, middle and ring fingers in a rotatory movement (see Figs.9-1, 2). It is usually applied to Feishu, Tanzhong, Rugen and Zhongwan

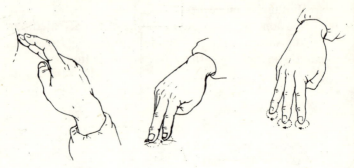

Fig.9 (1) Finger rotatory kneading

Fig.9 (2) Finger rotatory kneading

points.

Palm edge rotatory kneading The operator kneads a given part or point of a patient with his lower palm edge in a rotatory movement (see Fig.10).

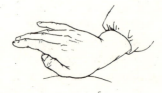

Fig.10 Palm edge rotatory kneading

Lower palm rotatory kneading The operator kneads a given part or point of a patient with his lower palm in a rotatory movement (see Fig.11). It is usually applied to the middle chest or navel.

6) Pinching manoeuvre

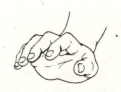

Fig.11 Lower palm rotatory kneading

The operator presses a point with his thumbnail (see Fig.12) with gradually increasing force. The skin should not be cut. After pressing, knead the part to relieve pain. It is mostly used in the treatment of infantile diseases, and applied to the seven points, including Tianting, Chengjiang, Laolong, Ershanmen, Weiling and Jingning.

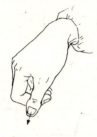

Fig.12 Pinching manoeuvre

7) Kneading manoeuvre

The operator presses hard on the patient's limbs and lower back with his palm and makes quick rotatory movements (see Fig.13).

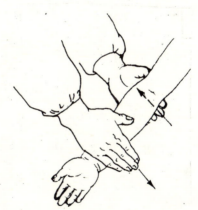

Fig.13 Kneading manoeuvre

8) Circular pushing manoeuvre

The operator pushes the selected points with his thumb or middle finger with a circular movement (see

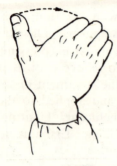

Fig.14 Circular pushing manoeuvre

Fig.14). In the process light force is used with slow frequency. Only the superficial part of the body is pushed instead of the deeper muscles. The movement frequency is about 80-120 cycle/min.

9) Lifting manoeuvre

Using the thumb and index finger or the second segment of the index and middle fingers, the operator grips the skin of the body and lifts it repeatedly (see Fig.15)

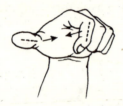

Fig.15 Lifting manoeuvre

until cyanosis appears.

10) Beating manoeuvre

The operator taps the points with his middle

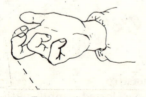
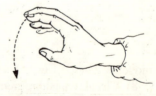

Fig.16 Tapping the points with the middle finger

Fig.17 Tapping the points with the middle finger

finger (see Figs.16 and 17). This is most often used on Yujijiao to relieve upward staring of eyes due to convulsions.

11) Shaking manoeuvre

The operator holds the ends of the bones forming the joint and moves them in a circular fashion (see Fig.18). This is usually applied to the neck and large joints of the limbs. The shaking increases gradually in extent and rate.

12) Spinal kneading and squeezing-kneading

Spinal kneading With the patient lying prostrate, the operator starts to grip and knead the skin in the lumbosacrum with

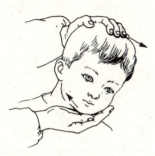

Fig.18 Shaking manoeuvre

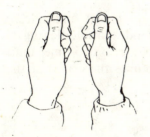

Fig.19(1) Spinal kneading

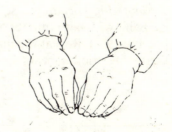

Fig.19(2) Spinal kneading

his thumbs and index fingers (see Figs.19-1,2). Do the operation upward along the spine (lifting once for

33

every three kneads) to the area of Dazhui (see Fig.19-3). Then rub with the middle finger along both sides of the spine back to the lumbosacrum. Repeat the whole operation 3 to 5 times.

This manoeuvre is effective for infantile indigestion, loss of appetite or sprains of the back, insomnia due to neuraasthenia, hypertension, and costal neuralgia in

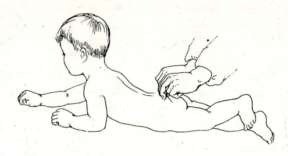

Fig.19 (3) Spinal kneading

adults.

Squeezing-kneading Squeeze, knead and release the point with both thumbs and index or middle fingers (see Fig.19-4). Repeat the manoeuvre 3 to 5 times until local congestion appears. Sometimes the centre of the

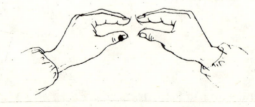

Fig.19 (4) Squeezing-kneading

point should be cut with a three-edged needle to induce a small amount of bleeding before the manipulation follows. It can clear away heat, and relieve inflammation and pain.

IV. Points Frequently Used in Infantile Tuina Therapy

Although the points used in infantile tuina therapy are not as numerous as those used in acupuncture, about one hundred points are selected (see Figs.20 and 21). Different schools lay particular emphasis on the points they consider the best.

Most of the eighty points described in this book are particular to infants except a few distributed in the fourteen meridians or extra points. These special points are located on the head, face, hand, foot, and especially in the palm and dorsum of the hand, and are described by dots, lines or areas.

1. Points on the Head and Face (see Fig.22)

1) Baihui

Location: On the midpoint of the line connecting the apexes of the two auricles.

Manipulation: Hold the forehead of the patient tightly with the left hand, press and knead the point 30 times (see Fig.23).

Action: Soothing the nerves, invigorating vital function.

Indications: Convulsions, infantile convulsions,

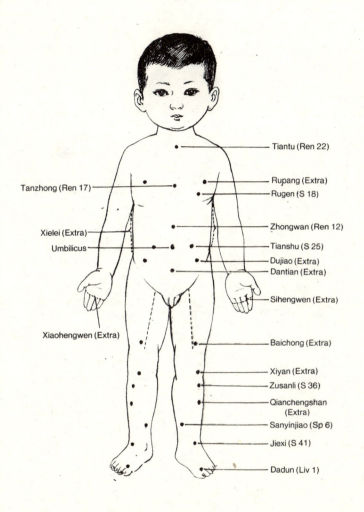

Fig.20 Commonly used tuina points in the front

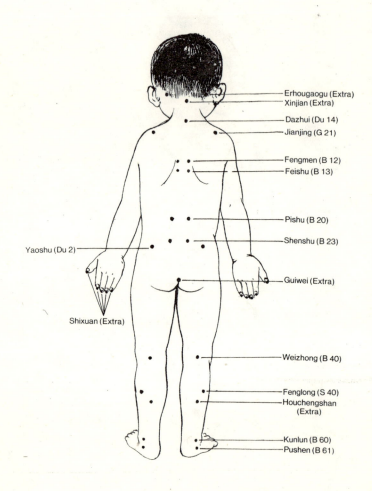

Fig.21 Commonly used tuina points on the back

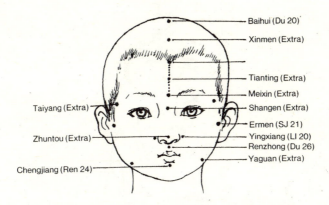

Fig.22 Points on the head and face

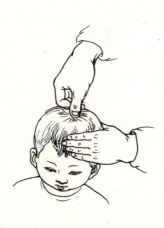

Fig.23 Pressing and kneading Baihui

headache, blurred vision, nasal obstruction, prolapsed rectum, bedwetting.

2) Xinmen (also called Xinfeng, Xinhui)

Location: 3 cun anterior to Baihui

Manipulation: Hold the head of the patient with two hands, repeat the pushing of the skin along the hairline to Xinmen (see Fig.24) 30 to 50 times.

Action: Soothing the nerves and resuscitation.

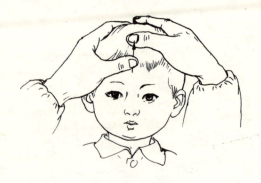

Fig.24 Pushing Xinmen

Indications: Convulsions, spasm, staring-up of the eyes, dizziness, blurred vision, nasal obstruction, rhinorrhea.

3) Zanzhu (also called Tianmen)

Location: On the medial extremity of the eyebrow.

Manipulation: Push along the skin from the part between eyebrows to the centre of the forehead. This is called "opening the heavenly door" (see Fig.25); push-

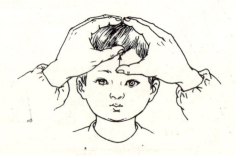

Fig.25 Pushing Zanzhu

ing straight to Xinmen is known as "opening the large heavenly door."

Action: Dispelling pathogenic wind from the exterior of the body, soothing the nerves and relieving headache.

Indications: Fever due to exogenous affection, headache, anhidrosis or little sweating, lassitude, fright.

4) Kangong

Location: 1 cun away from the eyebrow, directly above the pupil.

Manipulation: Press 1 cun away from the eyebrow with both thumbnails, then repeatedly push the skin from the middle of the eyebrows to the outer eyebrow ends (see Fig.26) 20 to 30 times.

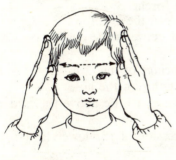

Fig.26 Pushing Kangong

Action: Inducing sweating and dispelling pathogenic factors from the exterior of the body, improving eyesight, relieving headache.

Indications: Exogenous affection and internal injury.

5) Taiyang

Location: in the depression about 1 cun posterior to the midpoint between the lateral end of the eyebrow and the outer canthus.

Manipulation: Massage the point with the thumb and middle finger (see Fig.27) 20 to 50 times. Forward massage is called the reinforcing method and backward

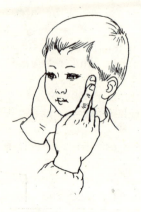

Fig.27 Massaging Taiyang

massage, the reducing method.

Action: Dispelling the pathogenic wind to relieve exogenous symptoms, removing heat and improving eye-sight, relieving pains.

Indications: Anhidrosis, hypohidrosis, hidrosis, chronic convulsions, exogenous affection and internal injury.

6) Pressing the points from Tianting to Chenjiang

Location:

Tianting—in the centre of the forehead

Meixin (glabella)—between the eyebrows

Zhigeng—below Meixin between the depression of eyes

Yannian—on the high bridge of the nose

Zhuntou (Suliao)—on the tip of the nose

Renzhong—below the nose, a little above the midpoint of the philtrum

Chenjiang—in the depression of the lower lip (see Fig.28-1)

Manipulation: Hold the patient's head with the left hand and press the seven points one after another with the right thumb nail (see Fig.28-2). Each point is pressed 3 to 5 times.

Action: Resuscitation, relieving convulsions.

Indications: Acute convulsions, loss of consciousness, exogenous affection of pathogenic wind and cold.

7) Huangfengrudong (A wasp entering cave)

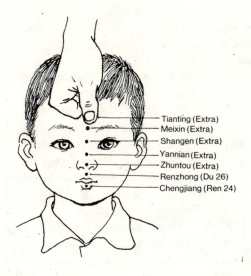

Fig.28 (1) Pressing the points from Tianting to Chenjiang

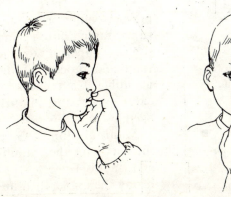

Fig.28 (2) Pressing Renzhong

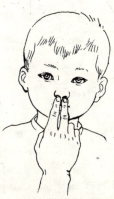

Fig.29 Huangfengrudong

Location: Near the nostrils

Manipulation: Hold the patient's head with the left hand and massage the inner nostrils or Yingxiang 20 to 30 times (see Fig.29).

Action: Inducing sweating and dispelling pathogenic factors from the exterior of the body, reducing fever.

Indications: Common cold, fever, nasal obstruction.

8) Yaguan (also called Jiache)

Location: One finger-breadth anterior and superior to the lower angle of the mandible where the masseter attaches at the prominence of the muscle when the teeth are clenched.

Manipulation: Press the points with the middle finger 5 times (see Fig.30) and knead them 30 times.

Indications: Trismus, facial paralysis.

9) Ermen (also called Fengmen)

Location: In the depression anterior to the supratragic notch and slightly superior to the condyloid process of the mandible. The point is located with the mouth open.

Manipulation: Grip the ears with the thumbs and index fingers, first lifting them and then applying the circular pushing manoeuvre (see

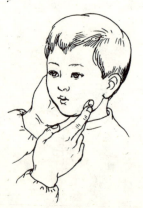

Fig.30 Pressing and kneading Yaguan

Fig.31) 30 times.

Indications: Convulsions, facial paralysis, tinnitus, deafness, toothache.

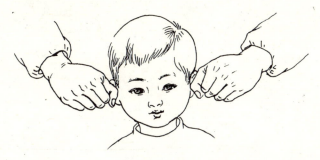

Fig.31 Fengmen

10) Qiaogong

Location: On either side of the neck, to the musculus sternocleido-mastoideus forming a straight line.

Manipulation: Hold the patient's head with one hand and apply the rotatory kneading manoeuvre with the other 30 times, or rub downwards as Fig.32 shows 50 times.

Indications: Infantile muscular torticollis, rigidity of the neck.

11) Erhougaogu (also called Erhou, Erji)

Location: In the depression at the posterior margin of the processus mastoideus, entering the hairline behind the ear.

Manipulation: Hold the patient's forehead with both hands. Knead the points with both thumbs 20 to 50 times (see Fig.33).

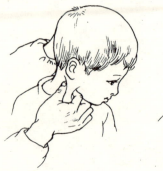
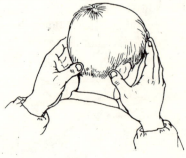

Fig.32 Kneading and rubbing Qiaogong

Fig.33 Kneading Erhougaogu

Action: Dispelling pathogenic wind from the exterior of the body, removing restlessness.

Indications: Common cold, headache, fever.

2. Points on the Back

1) Xinjian

Location: Between the second and third cervical vertebrae, below Yamen.

Manipulation: Press the point from the outside to the centre with both thumbs, index and middle fingers (see Fig.34). Sometimes a three-edged needle is used to prick the skin to draw blood, and then the manipulation is applied until local congestion appears.

Action: Eliminating accumulated heat, clearing the throat, anti-inflammation, relieving pain.

Indications: Sore throat, acute laryngoparalysis, acute tonsillitis, edema of vocal cords, hoarseness.

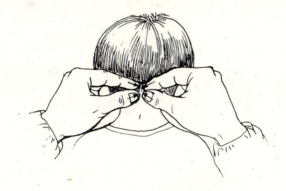

Fig.34 Pressing and kneading Xinjian

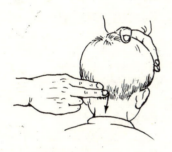

Fig.35 Pushing Tianzhu

2) Tianzhu

Location: Along the line from Dazhui upward to the back hairline.

Manipulation: Repeatedly push the skin downward to Dazhui (see Fig.35). 100 to 200 times with the pad of the right middle finger.

Action: Promoting downward flow of qi.

Indications: Vomiting, rigidity of the neck, headache due to common cold.

3) Dazhui

Location: Between the spinous processes of the seventh cervical vertebra and the first thoracic vertebra, approximately at the level of the shoulder.

Manipulation: Knead the point with the right thumb or middle finger (see Fig.36) 100 times.

Action: Removing exogenous affection and heat

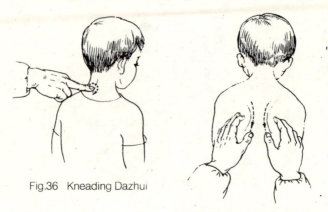

Fig.36 Kneading Dazhui

Fig.37 (2) Pushing Feishu

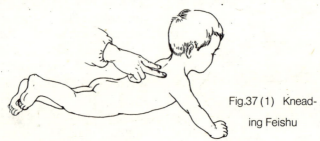

Fig.37 (1) Kneading Feishu

from the heart and lungs.

Indications: Common cold, rigidity of the neck, pain of the shoulder and back, fever, vomiting.

4) Feishu

Location: 1.5 cun lateral to the lower border of the spinous process of the third thoracic vertebra.

Manipulation: Repeatedly knead the point with the thumb or index or middle finger (see Fig.37-1) 50 to 100 times, or push the skin downward along the border of the scapula (see Fig.37-2) 100 to 300 times.

Action: Regulating qi of the lungs, removing deficiency, stopping coughing.

Indications: Asthma, cough, wheezing due to profuse phlegm, stuffiness of the chest, chest pain, fever.

5) Jizhu

Location: A straight line from lumbosacrum to Dazhui.

Manipulation: Push the skin forcefully with the pads of the index and middle fingers from Dazhui downward to the lumbosacrum (see Fig.38) 300 to 500 times, or tap the skin from Dazhui to the lumbosacrum until congestion appears.

Action: Regulating yin and yang, qi and blood, harmonizing the zang-fu organs and promoting smooth functioning of the meridians.

Indications: Fever, convulsions, night crying of babies, malnutrition, diarrhoea, vomiting, abdominal pain, constipation.

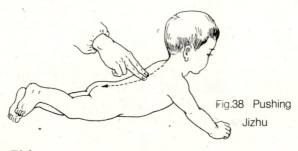

Fig.38 Pushing Jizhu

6) Pishu

Location: 1.5 cun lateral to the lower border of the spinal process of the eleventh thoracic vertebra.

Manipulation: Knead the point with the thumb or

middle finger 50 to 100 times.

Action: Strengthening the spleen and stomach, promoting digestion and removing dampness.

Indications: Vomiting, malnutrition, chronic convulsions, weak limbs.

7) Qijiegu

Location: A straight line from coccyx to the fourth lumbar vertebra.

Manipulation: Push the skin with the index and middle fingers from either direction (see Fig.39) 100 to 300 times.

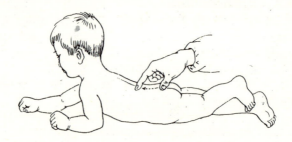

Fig.39 Pushing Qijiegu

Action: Warming yang and stopping diarrhoea by the reinforcing method (upward movement), reducing heat and stopping diarrhoea by the reducing method (downward movement).

Indications: Diarrhoea, dysentery, prolapsed rectum, constipation.

8) Guiwei

Location: At the tip of the coccyx.

Manipulation: Knead the point repeatedly 300 to

500 times with the thumb (see Fig.40) or knead the navel simultaneously for better results. Cupping is applied to the point in the treatment of diarrhoea and abdominal pain.

Action: Warming up yang and stopping diarrhoea.

Indications: Diarrhoea, abdominal pain, dysentery, prolapsed rectum.

9) Changqiang

Location: Midway between the tip of the coccyx and the anus.

Manipulation: Place the patient in a prone position and knead the point with the middle finger 50 to 100 times (see Fig.41).

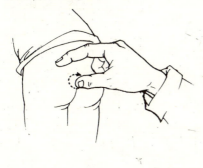

Fig.40 Kneading Guiwei

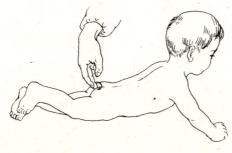

Fig.41 Kneading Changqiang

Action: Regulating the function of the intestines to counter inflammation.

Indications: Enteritis, diarrhoea, hemorrhoids, prolapsed rectum.

3. Points in the Thoracic and Costal Regions

1) Tiantu

Location: In the centre of the suprasternal fossa.

Manipulation: Hold the patient's head with the left hand and knead the point with the right middle finger 20 to 30 times (see Fig.42), or push and squeeze from the outside towards the centre of the point until local congestion appears (see Fig.43).

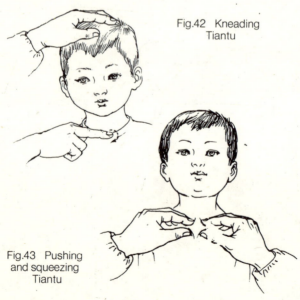

Fig.42 Kneading Tiantu

Fig.43 Pushing and squeezing Tiantu

Action: Obstruction by phlegm.

Indications: Dyspnea, sore throat, hoarseness.

2) Shanzhong

Location: On the middle of the sternum, between the nipples.

Manipulation: Push the skin from the centre of the point to the nipples with both thumb pads (see Fig.44-1) 30 to 60 times, or knead the point with the middle finger or push the skin from the manubrium sterni to the point with the index and middle fingers (see Fig.44-2) 30 to 60 times.

Action: Regulating qi of the lungs, stopping coughing.

Indications: Stuffiness of the chest, asthma, cough, vomiting, nausea.

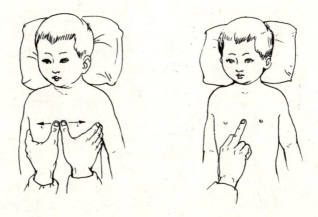

Fig.44 (1) Pushing Shanzhong   Fig.44 (2) Kneading Shanzhong

3) Rugen

Location: In the intercostal space, one rib below the nipple.

Manipulation: Knead the point with the middle finger or thumb 30 times.

Action: Regulating qi of the lungs, removing cough and phlegm.

Indications: Asthma, cough, stuffiness of the chest.

4) Xielei

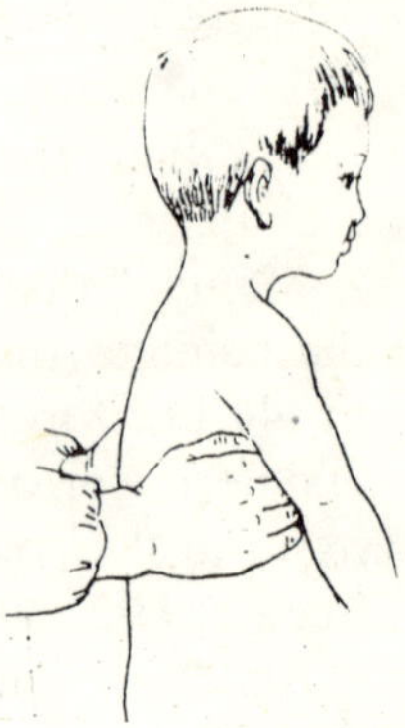

Location: At the place from below the costal regions to Tianshu.

Fig.45 Rubbing Xielei

Manipulation: Rub the place between the costal regions and Tianshu quickly 50 to 100 times (see Fig.45).

Action: Regulating qi flow and resolving phlegm.

Indications: Indigestion, stuffiness of the chest and abdominal distension due to the accumulation of phlegm.

5) Fuyinyang

Location: In the upper abdomen.

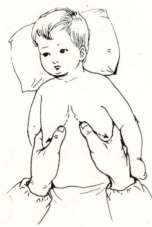

Fig.46 Pushing Fuyinyang

Manipulation: Push the skin with both thumbs forcefully along the costal margin outwards or from Zhongwan to the navel (see Fig.46) 100 to 200 times.

Action: Strengthening the stomach and spleen, and promoting digestion.

Indications: Abdominal pain and distension, indigestion, vomiting, nausea.

6) Zhongwan (also called Weiwan, Taicang)

Location: On the middle of the abdomen, 4 cun above the umbilicus.

Manipulation: Knead the point with the right palm or the index, middle and ring fingers (see Fig.47-1), or push the skin from Tiantu to Zhongwan or vice versa (see Fig.47-2) 30 to 50 times.

Action: Strengthening the spleen and stomach, and promoting digestion.

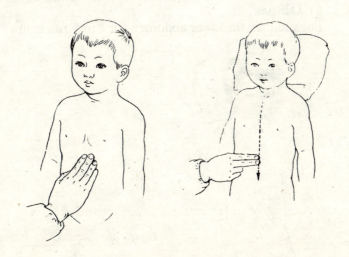

Fig.47(1) Kneading Zhongwan   Fig.47(2) Pushing Zhongwan

Indications: Abdominal distension, indigestion, vomiting, diarrhoea, loss of appetite, belching.

7) Duqi (also called Shenjue)

Location: In the navel.

Manipulation: Knead the navel with the index, middle and ring fingers (see Fig.48) 100 to 500 times. Clockwise kneading is known as the reinforcing method and counterclockwise kneading the reducing method.

Action: Warming up yang, and removing deficiency, strengthening the spleen to relieve diarrhoea.

Indications: Diarrhoea due to weakening function of the spleen, indigestion, abdominal distension, gurgling sound (reinforcing). Constipation, indigestion, abdominal distension, abdominal pain (reducing).

8) Dantian

Location: In the lower abdomen (or 2 to 3 cun below

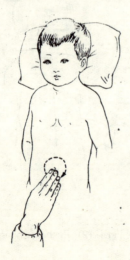

Fig.48 Kneading Duqi

the umbilicus).

Manipulation: Knead the point with the right palm or index finger (see Figs. 49-1,2) 100 to 300 times.

Action: Strengthening the kidneys.

Indications: Diarrhoea, abdominal pain, enuresis, prolapsed rectum, hernia.

9) Dujiao

Location: 2 cun below the umbilicus and 2 cun away from the tendinomuscles.

Manipulation: Pull both sides of the lateral abdominal tendinomuscles forcefully with the thumb, index and middle fingers. Frequent pulling of the tendinomuscles is known as "pulling Dujiao" (see Fig.50). Repeat the pulling of the tendinomuscles 5 to 6 times.

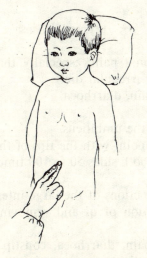

Fig.49 (1) Kneading Dantian

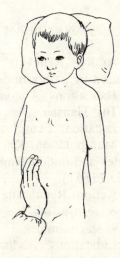

Fig.49 (2) Kneading Dantian with the palm

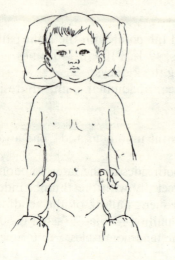
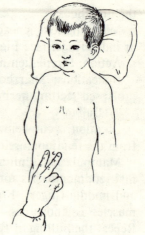

Fig.50 Kneading Dujiao   Fig.51 Kneading Tianshu

Action: Relieving abdominal pain, especially that caused by pathogenic cold or irregular diet.

Indications: Abdominal pain, diarrhoea.

10) Tianshu

Location: 2 cun lateral to the umbilicus.

Manipulation: Knead the point with the tips of the index and middle fingers on both sides 50 to 100 times (see Fig.51).

Action: Regulating the functions of the large intestine, readjusting the circulation of qi and removing food stagnation.

Indications: Abdominal pain, diarrhoea, constipation, abdominal distension, indigestion caused by food stagnation.

4. Points in the Medial Aspect of the Upper Limb and Palm (See Fig.52)

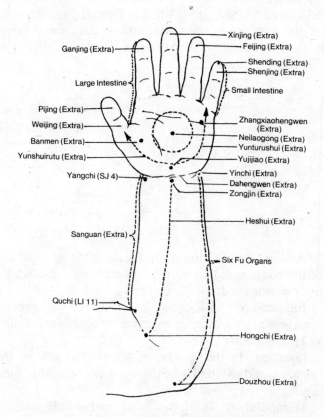

Fig.52 Points in the medial aspect of the upper limb and palm

1) Sanguan

Location: On the radial border of the forearm, on the line between the root of the palm and the radial end of the cubital crease.

Manipulation: Hold the index and middle fingers together and push along the line from the radial aspect of the wrist up to the radial end of the cubital crease with the pads of the two fingers 100 to 500 times (see Fig.53).

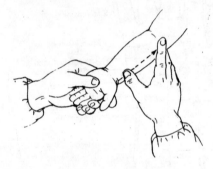

Fig.53 Pushing Sanguan

Action: Reinforcing qi and strengthening the yang of the body, and dispersing pathogenic cold and relieving exterior syndromes.

Indications: Abdominal pain, diarrhoea, general weakness after a disease, aversion to cold, weak limbs.

2) Tianheshui

Location: In the middle of the medial side of the forearm, midway between the wrist crease and cubital crease.

Manipulation: Hold the index and middle fingers together. Push with the pads of the fingers from transverse crease of the wrist straight up to the cubital crease 100 to 500 times (see Fig.54).

Action: Clearing pathogenic heat, relieving exterior symptoms and reducing pathogenic fire.

Indications: Febrile diseases, fever caused by common cold, tidal fever, excessive internal heat, irritability, restlessness, thirst, playing tongue, stiffness of tongue, convulsions.

3) Liufu

Location: At the ulna side, on the line between Yangchi to the elbow.

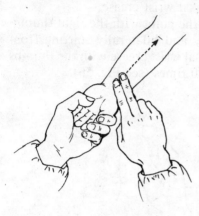

Fig.54 Pushing Tianheshui

Manipulation: Hold the index and middle fingers together. Push from the elbow joint straight to the root of the palm with the pads of the two fingers 100 to 500 times (see Fig.55).

Action: Clearing heat, cooling the blood, and detoxication.

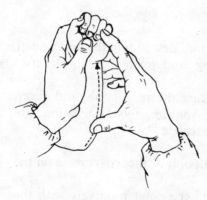

Fig.55 Pushing Liufu

Indications: High fever, irritability, dry stools, thirst preferring cold drinks, any other febrile diseases.

4) Dahengwen

Location: On the dorsal wrist crease.

Manipulation: Press the point with the right thumbnail, or push outwardly and bilaterally starting from the midpoint of the dorsal wrist crease with the thumbs of both hands 100 to 500 times (see Fig. 56).

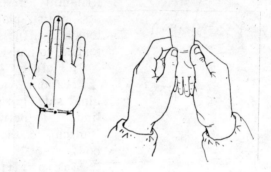

Fig.56 Pushing Dahengwen

Action: Expelling wind, descending the perverse qi, balancing yin and yang, and removing stagnation of food.

Indications: Vomiting, alternate chills and fever, asthma with excessive sputum, food stagnation, abdominal distension, diarrhoea.

5) Zongjin

Location: At the midpoint of the wrist crease on the palmar aspect.

Manipulation: Knead the point rotatively with the middle finger or thumb of the right hand or knead from the upper part down to Zongjin 20 to 30 times. Finish the manipulation by pressing heavily on this point (see Fig.57).

Action: Dispersing accumulated heat, antispasmotism, and easing the mind.

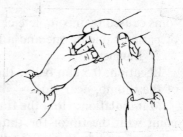
Fig.57 Kneading Zongjin

Indications: Convulsions, mental stress, diarrhoea, vomiting, mouth ulcers.

6) Yujijiao (also called Xiaotianxin)

Location: On the juncture between the major and minor thenar muscles, in the middle of the radial end of the wrist crease of the palmar aspect.

Manipulation: Hold the finger of the child with the left hand and press several times with the right thumbnail, then knead or tap the point 7 to 8 times with the dorsal aspect of the second phalangeal joint of the middle finger 100 to 300 times (see Fig.58).

Action: Removing the obstruction of orifices and eliminating stasis, stopping convulsions and easing the mind, brightening the eyes and clearing pathogenic heat.

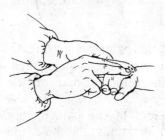
Fig.58 Kneading Yujijiao

Indications: Convulsions, epilepsy, blurred vision, redness, pain and swelling of the eye, excessive lacrimation, and symptoms caused by incomplete closing of infantile fontanel of patients one or one and a half years old.

7) Banmen

Location: 0.5 cun below the second phalangeal joint of the thumb, near Yuji.

Manipulation: Hold the fingers of the child. Rub the point with the tip of the thumb of the right hand, or rub back and forth on the surface of the major thenar muscle 100 to 300 times (see Fig.59).

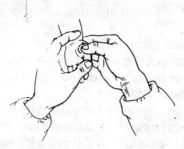

Fig.59 Kneading Banmen

Action: Relieving convulsions, removing food stagnation and promoting digestion, reducing excess heat of the spleen and stomach.

Indications: Acute or chronic convulsions, opisthotonus, indigestion.

8) Fenyinyang

Location: On the root of the palmar wrist crease, from the centre of Yujijiao, separating the major thenar muscle (Yangchi) and the minor thenar muscle (Yinchi).

Manipulation: Fix both sides of the palmar root with the index fingers of both hands and hold the dorsum of the patient's hand. Then push the muscles

200 to 300 times from the centre towards the outside with the pads of the thumbs of both hands (see Fig.60).

Action: Balancing yin and yang of the body, and regulating the functions of the zang-fu organs.

Indications: Diarrhoea, vomiting, fright, convulsions.

9) Hengwen to Banmen

Location: From the wrist transverse crease to the major thenar muscle.

Manipulation: Hold the patient's hand and push from the wrist transverse crease to Banmen (see Fig.61) 100 to 300 times.

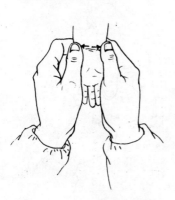

Fig.60 Fenyinyang

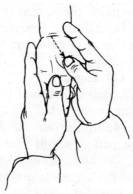

Fig.61 Hengwen to Banmen

Action: Relieving stuffiness of the chest and clearing heat of the stomach.

Indications: Stuffiness of the chest, vomiting.

10) Banmen to Hengwen

Location: From the second phalangeal joint of the thumb, via the major thenar muscle, to the wrist transverse crease.

Manipulation: Hold the patient's hand with the left hand. Push from Banmen down to the wrist transverse crease (see Fig.62) about 100 to 300 times.

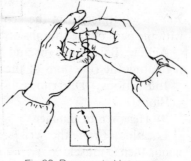
Fig.62 Banmen to Hengwen

Action: Building up the spleen and harmonizing the stomach.

Indications: Diarrhoea caused by a deficiency of spleen-yang.

11) Bagua

Location: Around Laogong in the palm.

Manipulation: Hold the patient's four fingers of the left hand with the palm facing upward. Press tightly between the second and the third phalangometacarpal joints with the thumb of the right hand. Then starting from the second phalangometacarpal joint, rotate clockwise or counterclockwise around the border of Laogong 100 to 500 times (see Fig.63).

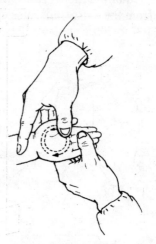
Fig.63 Kneading Neibagua

Action: Regulating and removing the obstruction of the circulation of qi and blood, and harmonizing the five zang organs.

Indications: Cough, diarrhoea, abdominal distension, food stagnation.

12) Neilaogong

Location: In the centre of the palm. When the fingers are flexed, the point is between the second and third metacarpal bones where the index and middle fingers point to.

Manipulation: Hold the patient's right hand with the left hand. Knead Neilaogong rotatively about 30 to 100 times with the tip of right index finger or thumb (see Fig.64).

Action: Clearing heat, relieving exterior syndromes, and stopping convulsions.

Indications: Convulsions caused by fright, fever due to common cold, all the Shi-heat symptoms.

13) Pijing

Location: At the radical side of the thumb from the tip of the thumb to its root along the margin between the red and white skin.

Manipulation: Hold the patient's left wrist in between the operator's index and middle fingers. Then push upward with the tip of the right thumb (reinforcing method). Pushing straight downward is known as the reducing method (see Figs. 65-1,2). Flexing the thumb and pushing leftward is also Reinforcing Method. Repeat the above pushing methods about 300 to 500 times.

Action: Building up the spleen and strengthening the stomach by the reinforcing method, and removing food stagnation and promoting digestion by the reducing method.

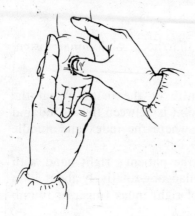

Fig.64 Kneading Neilaogong

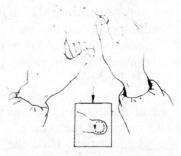

Fig.65 (1) Pushing Pijing

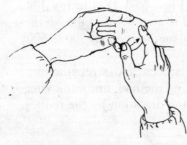

Fig.65 (2) Flexing the thumb and pushing Pijing

Indications: Weakness of the spleen and stomach, anorexia, emaciation, listlessness.

14) Dachang

Location: At the medial aspect, forming a straight line from the tip of the index finger to the finger web between the first and second metacarpal bones.

Manipulation: Hold the patient's other fingers tightly with the left hand. Pushing about 100 to 500 times from the tip of the index finger straight down to the finger web between the thumb and index finger is called reinforcing Dachang (see Fig.66). Pushing upward is reducing Dachang.

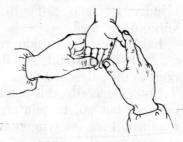

Fig.66 Pushing Dachang

Action: Regulating the functions of the intestines by the reinforcing method. Clearing heat from the large intestine and relaxing the bowels by the reducing method.

Indications: Diarrhoea, dysentery, constipation, abdominal pain.

15) Ganjing

Location: On the palmar surface, forming a straight line from the tip to the root of the index finger.

Manipulation: Push the pads of the patient's index finger about 100

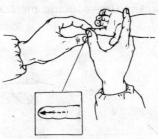

Fig.67 Pushing Ganjing

to 500 times from the root to its tip (see Fig.67).

Action: Clearing the heat from the Liver and Gallbladder Meridians, easing the mind and relieving convulsions.

Indications: Convulsion, redness of the eyes, anxiety, restlessness, fright, irritability and feverish sensations in the palms and soles.

Note: Generally, this point should be appropriately reduced, but not be reinforced. If it is necessary to reinforce it for the symptoms caused by insufficiency of the liver, then Shenjing can be treated instead of Ganjing. Some doctors use the reinforcing method to treat mumps.

16) Xinjing

Location: On the palmar surface, forming a straight line from the tip to the root of the middle finger.

Manipulation: Hold the patient's palm with the left hand. Push from the tip to the root of the middle finger or vice versa with the thumb pad about 100 to 500 times. Upward pushing is called reinforcing Xinjing, and downward pushing, reducing Xinjing (see Fig.68).

Note: Some have said that upward pushing on this point is the reducing method, and pushing rotatively,

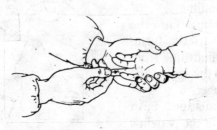

Fig.68 Pushing Xinjing

the reinforcing method. Or only the reducing method is applied to this point, the reinforcing method not being suitable. If Xinjing needs to be reinforced, the pushing method can be applied to Tianheshui instead.

17) Feijing

Location: On the palmar surface of the ring finger and a little bit lateral to the ulna aspect, forming a straight line from the root to the tip of the ring finger.

Manipulation: Hold the tip of the patient's ring finger with the left hand, and put the palm upward. Push from the root of the ring finger straight up to the tip with the pads of the right thumb (see Fig.69) about 100 to 500 times. Pushing the same number of times contrarily downward is called reinforcing the lungs.

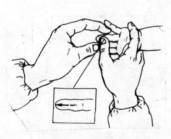

Fig.69 Pushing Feijing

Action: Tonifying qi of the lung by the reinforcing method and expelling excessive heat from the lung by the reducing method.

Indications: Common cold, cough, asthma with excessive sputum, constipation.

18) Shenjing

Location: On the palmar aspect of the little finger and a little bit inclined to the ulnar aspect, forming a straight line from the tip to the root of the little finger.

Manipulation: Push along the line from the tip to the root of the little finger with the tip of the right thumb about 100 to 500 times (see Fig.70). This is called reducing Shenjing. Pushing straight up to the tip of the little finger is named reinforcing Shenjing.

Action: Nourishing the kidney and strengthening the yang of the body by the reinforcing method, and purging the stagnated heat for the lower Jiao by the reducing method.

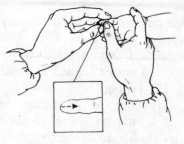

Fig.70 Pushing Shenjing

Indications: Congenital deficiency, weakness after chronic disease, morning diarrhoea, enuresis, cough, asthma.

19) Shending

Location: At the tip of the little finger.

Manipulation: Knead the point with the tip of the middle finger or thumb (see Fig.71) about 100 to 500 times.

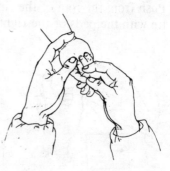

Fig.71 Kneading Shending

Action: Astringing the primary qi of the body, strengthening the exterior of the body and stopping perspiration.

Indications: Spontaneous sweating, night sweating, delayed closure of the fontanel.

20) Xiaochangjing

Location: On the ulnar border of the little finger,

forming a straight line from the tip to the root of the finger.

Manipulation: Push from the tip to the root of the small finger along its ulnar aspect (see Fig.72) with the belly of the right thumb about 100 to 500 times. This is the reinforcing method. Downward pushing is the reducing method.

Action: Clearing heat and diauresis by the reducing method. If there is pathogenic heat in the heart meridian to be further shifted to the small intestine, the reducing method can be used on this point and Qingheshui in order to strengthen the action of clearing the heat and diauresis.

Indications: Diarrhoea, scanty urine, anuria, high fever, afternoon fever.

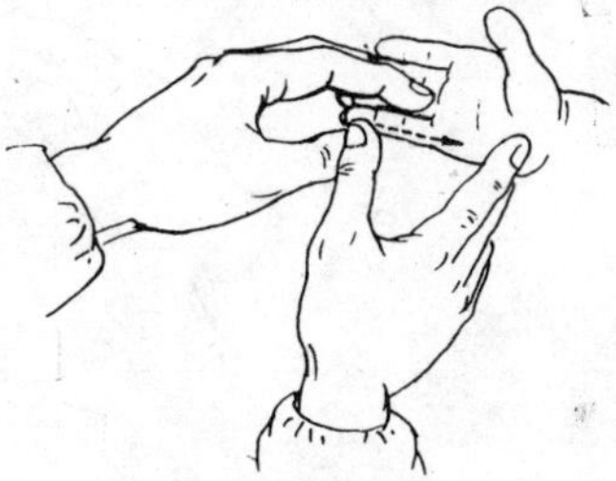

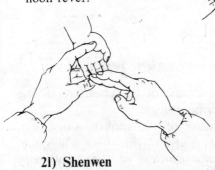

Fig.72 Pushing Xiaochangjing

Fig.73 Kneading Shenwen

21) Shenwen

Location: At the palmar aspect, on the transverse crease of the root of the little finger.

Manipulation: Press and knead Shenwen with the tip of the middle finger or thumb about 100 to 500 times (see Fig.73).

Action: Expelling wind, brightening the eyesight, dispersing lumps and stagnations.

Indications: Redness of the eyes, thrush, diseases caused by heat poison.

22) Xiaohengwen

Location: On the transverse creases of the phalango-metacarpal joints of the index, middle, ring and little fingers.

Manipulation: Press tightly with the thumbnail 3 to 5 times. Or push laterally along the transverse creases of the fingers with the middle finger about 100 to 300 times (see Fig.74).

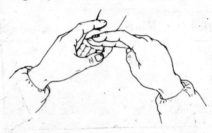

Fig.74 Pressing or pushing Xiaohengwen

Action: Relieving stiffness of the chest, removing stagnations and dissolving phlegm.

Indications: Ulceration of the mouth, salivation, cough with excessive sputum, trachitis, whooping, cough, pneumonia and disorders of the respiratory system.

23) Shuidilaoyue

Location: Along the border of the little finger from the tip, via the root of the palm to the centre where Neilaogong is located.

Manipulation: Hold the tips of the four fingers of the patient's left hand with the left hand. Pinch the wrist joint with the index and middle fingers of the right hand. Push along the lateral border from the tip through the root of the palm to Neilaogong (see Fig.75) with the radial aspect of the thumb about 100 to 500 times.

Action: Clearing pathogenic heat.

Indications: Accumulation of heat in the heart meridian and all heat syndromes.

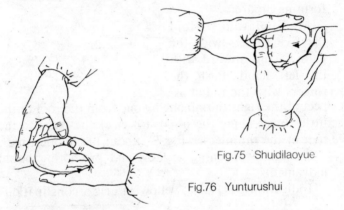

Fig.75 Shuidilaoyue

Fig.76 Yunturushui

24) Yunturushui

Location: From the tip of the thumb to the little finger, forming a curve.

Manipulation: Hold the patient's five fingers with the left hand. Let the palm face upward. Push with the radial aspect of the right thumb from the root of the thumb along the radial border of the palm to the tips of the remaining fingers, ending at the little finger about 100 to 300 times (see Fig.76). This is the manipulation of transporting earth into water.

Action: Clearing damp-heat from the stomach and reinforcing insufficiency of water.

Indications: Diarrhoea, abdominal distension, borborygomia, indigestion.

25) Yunshuirutu

Location: From the root of the little finger crossing the tips of the others to the thumb, forming an arc.

Manipulation: Hold the five fingers with the palm facing upward with the left hand. Push the fingers with the radial aspect of the right thumb one by one from the root of the little finger along the ulnar aspect of the palm to the root of the thumb (see Fig.77) about 100 to 300 times.

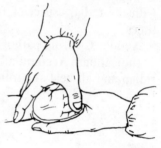

Fig.77 Yunshuirutu

Action: Moistening dryness and promoting bowel movements.

Indications: Dysuria, yellowish urine, constipation.

5. Points Along the Lateral Aspect of the Upper Limb and the Dorsum of the Palm (see Fig.78)

1) Yiwofeng

Location: In the depression of the middle of the wrist transverse crease on the dorsal aspect.

Manipulation: Hold the patient's hand with the left

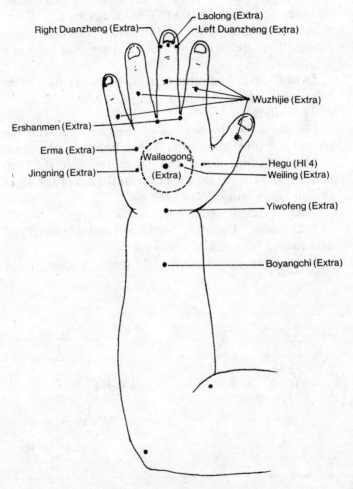

Fig.78 Points along the lateral aspect of the upper limb and the dorsum of the palm

hand. Then press the point with the tip of right thumb or index finger about 100 to 300 times (see Fig.79).

Action: Warming the middle jiao, promoting circulation of qi, relieving abdominal pain and stopping joint pain.

Indications: Abdominal pain, borborygmia, common cold, redness, swelling and joint pain.

2) Weiling

Location: On the dorsum of the hand between the second and third metacarpal bones, beside Wailaogong.

Manipulation: Press the point between the two bones 3 to 5 times (see Fig.80) with the tip of the right thumb. Then rub it after pressing.

Action: Resuscitation from coma.

Indications: Tinnitus, headache, and unconsciousness caused by acute convulsions.

Note: If an unconscious child makes a sound from

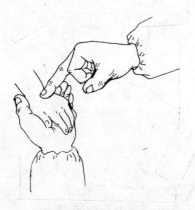

Fig.79 Pressing Yiwofeng

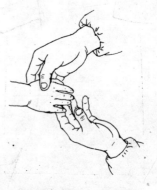

Fig.80 Pressing Weiling

the throat after pressing, the prognosis is better than if no sound is made. Therefore this manipulation can be used to judge the severity of a disease.

3) Jingning

Location: On the dorsum of hand beside Wailaogong, in the depression between the fourth and fifth metacarpal bones.

Manipulation: With the palm facing upward, hold the patient's ring finger between his left thumb and index finger, and stabilize the wrist between the right middle and index fingers. Then press the point with the right thumbnail 3 to 5 times, and knead it soon after the pressing (see Fig.81).

Action: Promoting the digestion of food and removing food stagnation.

Indications: Asthma with excessive sputum, retching, palpable lumps in the abdomen or fullness in the chest and abdomen.

4) Wailaogong

Location: In the centre of the dorsum of the hand, opposite Neilaogong, which is in the centre of the palm.

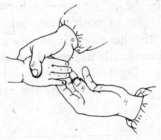

Fig.81 Pressing Jingning

Manipulation: Place the wrist in between the index and middle fingers of the left hand and hold the patient's fingers with the thumb, ring and little fingers for steadiness. Then knead the point with the tip of the right thumb or middle finger about 30 to 50 times (see Fig.82).

Action: Warming the yang of the body, dispersing pathogenic cold and warming the lower jiao.

Indications: Stool with undigested food, borborygmia, diarrhoea, dysentery due to cold attack, abdominal pain, hernia, prolapsed anus, ascariasis.

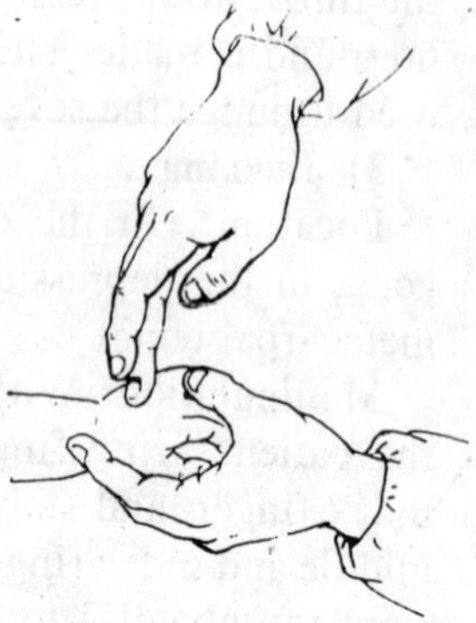

5) Ershanmen

Location: In the centre of the dorsum of the hand, in the depression between the third and fourth metacarpal bones.

Fig.82 Kneading Wailaogong

Manipulation: With the patient's palm downward, fix the patient's wrist between the index and middle fingers of both hands, and support the patient's palm with the ring fingers (see Fig.83-1). Then use both thumbnails to press the point tightly about 3 to 5 times (see Fig.83-2).

Action: Relieving the exterior syndromes by diaph-

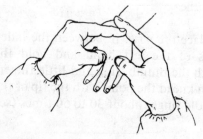

Fig.83 (1) Pressing Ershanmen

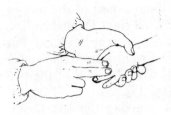

Fig.83 (2) Kneading Ershanmen

oresis, promoting smooth circulation of blood and qi to relax muscles and tendons.

Indications: Febrile symptoms caused by pathogenic wind or cold, anhidrosis, asthma with excessive sputum, stuffiness of the chest.

6) Laolong

Location: 0.1 cun posterior to the nail of the middle finger.

Manipulation: Hold the wrist with the left hand and pinch the middle finger forcefully between the right thumb and index finger. Then press the point with the thumbnail about 5 to 10 times (see Fig.84).

Action: Resuscitating an unconscious patient, stopping convulsions, reducing fever and the pathogenic fire.

Indications: Acute febrile convulsions, especially convulsions with the eyes looking upward, fever, irritability, fright, restlessness, afternoon fever, dull mind, wailing, trance.

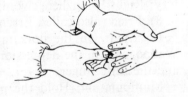

Fig.84 Pressing Laolong

7) Duanzheng

Location: On the margin between the red and white skin besides the root of the nail of the middle finger. The point at the radial side is called the left Duanzheng, and the point at the ulnar aspect of the root of the nail of the middle finger, the right Duanzheng.

Manipulation: Hold the wrist with the left hand. Put the middle finger between the right thumb and index finger, and press both points with the nails of the two fingers about 5 to 10 times (see Fig.85).

Action: Ascending qi by pressing the left Duan-

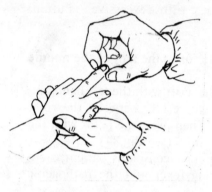

Fig.85 Pressing Duanzheng

zheng, descending qi by pressing the right Duanzheng.

Indications: Left Duanzheng: diarrhoea and dystentery; Right Duanzheng: vomiting and epistaxis.

8) Erma (also called Errenshangma)

Location: On the dorsum of the hand, lateral to Wailaogong, in the depression between the ring finger and the little finger.

Manipulation: Hold the patient's fingers with the left hand. Then rotate and knead the point about 100 to 300 times with the tip of right thumb or of the middle finger (see Fig.86).

Action: Nourishing and reinforcing yin of the kid-

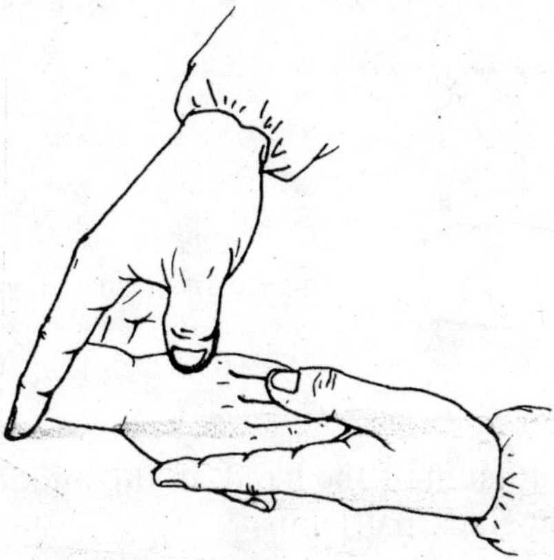

Fig.86 Kneading Erma

neys, and strengthening kidney yang.

Indications: Dysuria, indigestion, abdominal pain, weak body constitution, prolapsed rectum, enuresis, cough, asthma.

9) Tianmenruhukou

Location: Along the lateral side from the tip of the thumb to the place between the thumb and index finger.

Manipulation: Hold the patient's thumb with the left thumb and index finger. Then push from the tip of the thumb down to the intermetacarpal region between the thumb and index finger with the medial aspect of the right thumb about 100 to 300 times (see Fig.87).

Action: Smoothing the flow of qi and harmonizing blood circulation.

Indications: Anhidrosis, clenched teeth, sore throat, fullness of the chest.

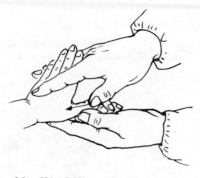

Fig.87 Pushing Tianmenhukou

10) Wuzhijie

Location: On the dorsum of the hand, in the middle of the five phalangometacarpal joints.

Manipulation: Hold the wrist with the left hand. Press forcefully into the five phalangometacarpal joints respectively with the right thumb and index finger that are opposite to each other on the dorsal and palmar aspect about 3 to 5 times (see Fig.88).

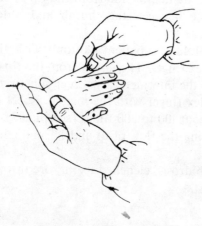

Fig.88 Pressing Wuzhijie

Action: Resuscitating an unconscious patient and stopping convulsions.

Indications: Convulsions and spasms.

11) Shixuan

Location: At the tips of all the fingers.

Manipulation: Hold the fingers with the left hand. Press respectively on the tips of all the fingers with the right thumbnail about 1 to 3 times (see Figs.89-1,2).

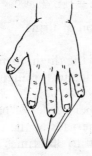 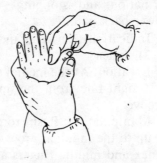

Fig.89 (1) Shixuan   Fig.89 (2) Pressing Shixuan

Action: Resuscitating an unconscious patient and reducing fever.

Indications: Acute convulsions, dull mind and morbid night crying of babies.

6. Points of the Lower Limbs

1) Zupangguang

Location: 6 cun above Xuehai, corresponding to the area of Jimen, pertaining to the Spleen Meridian of the Foot Taiyin.

(Note: The left point is the bladder and the right, Mingmen.)

Manipulation: Pinch the point with the thumb and index finger about 3 to 5 times (see Fig.90).

Action: Promoting urination and stopping lower back pain.

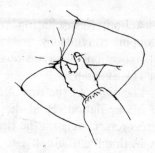

Fig.90 Pinching Zupangguang

Indications: Dysuria and retention of urine.

2) Jimen

Location: At the medial aspect of the thigh, forming a straight line from the upper border to the inguinal groove.

Manipulation: Push from the upper border of patella up to the inguinal groove with the pads of the right index and middle fingers about 100 to 300 times (see Fig.91).

Action: Mild property and remarkable diauretic action.

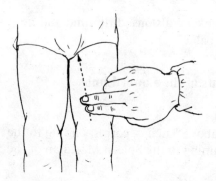

Fig.91 Pushing Jimen

Indications: Dysuria, yellowish urine, retention of urine, watery diarrhoea.

3) Xuehai (also called Baichong)

Location: 2.5 cun from the superior-medial aspect of the patella.

Manipulation: Press and knead the point with the belly of the right thumb about 30 times or pinch the point 3 to 5 times (see Fig.92).

Action: Removing obstruction of the meridians and stopping spasms.

Indications: Contracture of the four limbs, weakness and pain of the lower extremities.

4) Xiyan (also called Guiyan)

Location: In the two depressions below the patella.

Manipulation: Put the tips of the right thumb and index finger on the medial and lateral depressions below the patella (Neixiyan and Waixiyan). Then knead the two points forcefully and alternately about 10 to 15 times (see Fig.93).

Action: Stopping spasms and easing the mind.

Indications: Weakness and atrophy of the lower limbs,

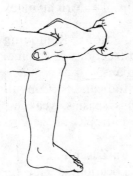

Fig.92 Pinching Baichong

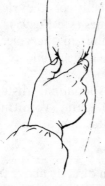

Fig.93 Pinching Xiyan

convulsions and spasms.

5) Weizhong

Location: A point of the Bladder Meridian of Foot-Taiyang, in the centre of the popliteal fossa and in the depression between the two tendons.

Manipulation: Hold the ankle joint with the left hand. Hook the point with the tip of the right index finger 5 to 10 times (see Fig.94).

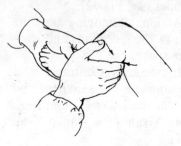

Fig.94 Pinching Weizhong

Action: Removing obstructions of the meridians.

Indications: Convulsions, spasms, weakness and atrophy of the lower limbs.

6) Zusanli

Location: 3 cun below Waixiyan and 1 cun lateral to the tibia.

Manipulation: Press or knead the point with the belly of the right thumb 5 to 10 times (see Fig.95).

Action: Building up the spleen, harmonizing the stomach and regulating qi of the middle jiao.

Indications: Abdominal distension, abdominal pain, vomiting, diarrhoea, weakness and atrophy of the lower limbs.

7) Sanyinjiao

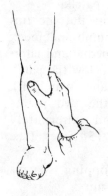

Fig.95 Pressing and kneading Zusanli

Location: 3 cun directly above the tip of the medial malleolus, pertaining to the Spleen Meridian of Foot Taiyin.

Manipulation: Press and knead the point or push downward from the point with the tip of the right thumb (see Fig.96).

Action: Removing obstructions of the meridians, activating the circulation of blood, regulating the function of the lower jiao, dispelling pathogenic damp heat, and readjusting the water passages.

Indications: Enuresis, retention of urine, frequent urination, painful urination.

8) Jiexi

Location: On the transverse crease anterior to the ankle, in the depression between the two tendons.

Manipulation: Press the point with the right thumb nail about 3 to 5 times, or knead the point with the tip of the thumb 50 to 100 times (see Fig.97).

Indications: Convulsions, constant diarrhoea and vomiting, motor impairment of the ankle joint.

9) Pushen

Location: In the depression inferior to the lateral malleolus.

Manipulation: Press or pinch the point with the

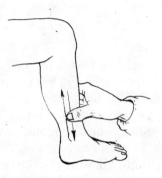

Fig.96 Pushing Sanyinjiao

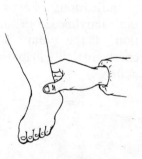

Fig.97 Pressing Jiexi

right thumb and index finger 3 to 5 times (see Fig.98).

Indications: Coma and convulsions.

10) Yongquan

Location: In the anterior depression of the sole of the foot.

Manipulation: Hold the patient's heel with the left hand. Press and knead the point with the belly of the right thumb 50 to 100 times (see Fig.99), or push from the point downward 100 to 300 times.

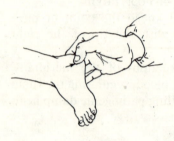

Fig.98 Pressing or pinching Pushen

Action: Conducting the fire downward, reducing fever due to deficiency of yin, and stopping vomiting by kneading on the left side and diarrhoea by kneading on the right side.

Indications: Fever, vomiting, diarrhoea, burning sensation of the palms, soles and chest, difficult urination, irritability.

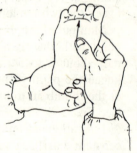

Fig.99 Kneading Yongquan

V. Indications of the Commonly Used Points and Prescriptions for Common Infantile Diseases

For the sake of study and clinical application, the indications of the commonly used points are classified as follows:

1. Dispelling the pathogenic factors from the exterior of the body: Push Zanzhu and Meigong, manipulate Taiyang and Erhougaogu by the reinforcing method, pinch Fengchi, squeeze and knead Xinjian and Dazhui, rub Yingxiang, massage Jianjing, push Sanguan and Tianheshui, and pinch and knead Ershanmen.

2. Reducing heat: Clear Ganjing, Xinjing, Pijing, Shenjing, Dachang, Xiaochang and Weijing. Push Tianheshui forward and Liufu backward. Pinch and knead Yujijiao and Neilaogong. Reduce Banmen, manipulate Neilaogong, pinch Sihengwen, push Xiaohengwen, knead Shenwen, push the spine, rub Yongquan and pinch Shixuan.

3. Tonification: Reinforce Pijing, Xinjing, Feijing, the kidneys, the large intestine and the small intestine. Knead Erma, Dantian, Shenshu, push Sanguan, rub Duqi by reinforcing, knead the spine, rub Zhongwan, pinch and knead Zusanli, and knead Feishu and Pishu.

4. Warming yang and dispelling cold: Pinch and knead Ershanmen and Yiwofeng. Knead Wailaogong, rub Duqi by reinforcing, push Sanguan, knead Dantian and rub Erma.

5. Digesting and removing stagnation: Clear and reinforce Pijing, clear Banmen, manipulate along Neibagua, divide yin and yang, knead Zhongwan to divide abdominal yin and yang. Rub Duqi for regulation, pinch and knead Zusanli and knead Pishu.

6. Stopping diarrhoea: Push the large intestine by reinforcing and Banmen forward to Hengwen. Manipulate the spleen and kidneys, and push them upward, press Houchengshan, pinch the left Duanzheng, knead Guiwei, push Qijiegu upward, knead the spine, rub Qiwei, push Qijie, rub Duqi, knead Tianshu, squeeze and knead Tianshu, massage Dujiao, knead and pinch Zusanli, and knead Yongquan.

7. Relieving abdominal pain: Massage Dujiao, pinch and knead Yiwofeng, massage Houchengshan, press and knead Shenshu.

8. Promoting defecation: Push the big intestine by the reducing method, pinch and knead the arm Yangchi, push and press Houchengshan downward, rub Duqi by reducing, push Qijiegu downward, knead Guiwei and manipulate along Neibagua.

9. Checking vomiting: Divide the abdominal yin and yang, push Tianzhu, manipulate Neibagua, push Hengwen forward to Banmen, clear Weijing and rub both the costal regions.

10. Promoting urination: Push and press Dantian, push Jimen, clear the small intestine, knead Yujijiao,

clear Shenjing, knead the arm Yangchi and pinch Chengjiang.

11. Regulating qi of the lungs, resolving phlegm and stopping cough: Push and knead Tanzhong, knead Rugen, Rupang and Feishu, clear Feijing, manipulate along Neibagua, squeeze and knead Tiantu, rub both the costal regions, knead and push the palmar Xiaohengwen.

12. Soothing the nerves: Push Zanzhu and Meigong, pinch Shangen and Yintang, pinch and knead Baihui, knead Yujijiao, pinch and knead Wuzhijie, clear Ganjing and Xinjing.

13. Resuscitating: Pinch and press Meigong, push Zanzhu, pinch Renzhong, Shixuan, Ershanmen, Jingning and Weiling.

14. Checking sweating: Knead Shending and manipulate Taiyang by reinforcing.

Prescriptions for Infantile Common Diseases:

1. Cold

Prescription 1: Push Zanzhu, Meigong, manipulate Taiyang, Erhougaogu, pinch Fengchi and knead Dazhui.

For wind-cold, add pushing Sanguan and kneading Ershanmen.

For wind-heat, add pushing Tianheshui and kneading Yujijiao.

For fever, add pushing Tianheshui and the spine.

For cough, add manipulation of Neibagua and clearing of Feijing.

Prescription 2: Clear Ganjing 10 times, Feijing 10 times, push Tianheshui 15 times, pinch Wuzhijie, push heavily Liufu 15 times, knead the spine and Dazhui.

2. Fever

1) For fever caused by exogeneous affection, see the prescriptions for cold.

2) Fever due to deficiency of yin:

Prescription: Knead Erma to strengthen Shenjing and Pijing, push Neibagua to divide yin and yang, push Tianheshui, pinch and knead Zusanli, knead Yongquan. Kneading Shending is added for night sweating.

3) Shi heat in the lungs and stomach:

Prescription: Clear Feijing and Weijing, push and clear the large intestine, push the spine, rub Duqi by the reducing method, pinch and knead Zusanli.

4) Fever caused by summer heat:

Prescription: Knead Yujijiao and Yiwofeng to tonify Shenjing, knead Erma to clear Banmen and divide yin and yang, push Tianheshui and knead Shenwen.

3. Cough

1) Cough caused by exogeneous pathogenic factors:

Prescription 1: Push Meigong, Zanzhu and Taiyang to clear Feijing, push along Neibagua, knead Tanzhong and Feishu. Pushing Xiaohengwen is added for open rale and kneading Xiaohengwen for moist rale.

Prescription 2: Push along Neibagua 10 to 15 times to clear Feijing and Ganjing 10 times, push Tianheshui 10 times.

2) Cough due to internal injury:

Prescription 1: Reinforce Pijing and Feijing, push along Neibagua, knead Tanzhong, Rugen, Rupang,

Feishu and the spine.

Prescription 2: Push against Neibagua, knead Erma, reinforce Pijing and Feijing.

4. Asthma

Prescription: Push against Neibagua to clear Feijing, push Xiaohengwen, knead Tanzhong, tap Tiantu (or squeeze and knead Tiantu), knead and rub both intercostal regions. Pushing Tianheshui is added for fever, Sanguan for fearing cold. Knead Yiwofeng. Erma is added for delicate constitution with chronic disease and failure of the kidneys to receive qi. Reinforce Shenjing and push Sanguan.

5. Pneumonia

Prescription 1: Push Pijing to clear Feijing and Ganjing, push Tianheshui, Neibagua and Xiaohengwen, knead the palmar Xiaohengwen, push and knead Tanzhong, knead Feishu, push the internal aspect of the scapula up and down.

Prescription 2: Knead Yujijiao and Yiwofeng, reinforce Shenjing, clear Banmen, push against Neibagua to clear Feijing, push Xiaohengwen, knead the palmar Xiaohengwen and push Tianheshui.

In the case of persistent fever, squeeze and knead both sides of Tiantu to the xiphoid process, both sides of Dazhui and the first lumbar vertebra until subcutaneous mild stasis appears.

Prescription 2: Push against Neibagua to clear Ganjing and Feijing, knead the palmar Xiaohengwen and push Liufu. In the case of convulsions due to high fever, tapping Yujijiao is added. For headache, kneading of Yangchi (3 cun directly above Yiwofeng) is added.

6. Abdominal distension
Prescription: Push Pijing, Banmen and Neibagua, knead Zhongwan to divide abdominal yin and yang, rub Duqi, press Pishu and knead Zusanli.

7. Diarrhoea
1) Diarrhoea due to abnormal diet:

Prescription 1: Push Pijing, Dachang, Banmen and Neibagua, knead Zhongwan to divide abdominal yin and yang, pinch and knead Zusanli.

Prescription 2: Push along Neibagua 10 times, clear Weijing 10 times, push Tianheshui 15 times and the small intestine 5 times.

2) Diarrhoea due to heat:

Prescription 1: Clear and reinforce Pijing and Weijing, push Dachang, and Tianheshui, clear Xiaochang, push Jimen, pinch and knead Yujijiao, rub Duqi and knead Zusanli.

Prescription 2: Push Liufu 15 times, clear Dachang, Pijing and Weijing 15 times, and push Qijiegu downward 10 times.

3) Diarrhoea due to cold:

Prescription 1: Push Sanguan, knead Wailaogong, reinforce Pijing, push Dachang and Qijiegu upward, knead Guiwei, rub Duqi for reinforcement, and pinch and knead Zusanli.

Prescription 2: Knead Wailaogong 20 times, clear Weijing, and push Tianheshui 10 times.

4) Diarrhoea due to deficiency of the spleen:

Prescription 1: Reinforce Pijing, push Dachang and Sanguan, manipulate along Neibagua, the kidneys and spleen, pinch the spine, push Qijiegu upward, knead Guiwei, rub Duqi for reinforcement, pinch and knead

Zusanli.

Prescription 2: For mild cases, knead Wailaogong 10 times, clear and reinforce Pijing 10 times, and clear Ganjing 5 times.

For severe cases, knead Erma 10 times, clear and reinforce Pijing 10 times and Dachang 15 times.

5) Diarrhoea caused by fright:

Prescription: Manipulate against Neibagua, push Dachang, Yunturushui, and the kidneys, push Qijiegu upward, knead Guiwei, push Sanguan, pinch Wuzhijie, Shixuan, Ershanmen and Laolong, pacify the liver or pinch and knead Yujijiao.

Note: The above five kinds of diarrhoea may be treated by cupping Guiwei for 3 to 5 minutes after massage. This method can also be applied independently. Most patients stop crying and fall asleep after cupping.

8. Dysentery

1) Dysentery with bloody stools:

Prescription 1: Divide yin and yang (with yin predominates), push Liufu backward, clear Xinjing and Dachang, push Tianheshui, pinch and knead Yujijiao, clear Feijing, rub Dujiao, pinch and knead Zusanli.

Prescription 2: Push Liufu backward 10 times, manipulate Neibagua 10 times, clear Dachang 15 times and Ganjing 5 times, and push Qijiegu downward 5 times.

2) Dysentery with white mucous stool:

Prescription 1: Divide yin and yang (when yang predominates), reinforce Pijing, push Sanguan, knead Wailaogong and Yiwofeng, push Dachang and Qijiegu upward, knead Erma, and pinch and knead Zusanli.

Prescription 2: Knead Wailaogong 10 times, clear and reinforce Dachang 15 times, and Pijing 10 times.

Pushing of Tianheshui is added for fever, and of Erma for delicate constitution.

9. Vomiting

1) Vomiting due to abnormal diet:

Prescription: Reinforce Pijing, manipulate against Neibagua and Banmen, clear Weijing to divide yin and yang, push Tianzhu, pinch and knead Zusanli.

2) Vomiting caused by heat:

Prescription: Reinforce Pijing, clear Weijing and Banmen, push Tianheshui, pinch and knead Yujijiao, push Tianzhu, and pinch and knead Zusanli.

3) Vomiting caused by cold:

Prescription: Reinforce Pijing, knead Wailaogong, manipulate against Neibagua, push Sanguan and Tianzhu, pinch and knead Zusanli, and knead Hegu.

10. Infantile malnutrition

Prescription 1: Knead the spine, manipulate along Neibagua, push Sanguan, pinch and knead Sihengwen, manipulate Banmen, rub Duqi, knead Zhongwan and Pishu, pinch and knead Zusanli.

Prescription 2: Knead Erma 15 times, reinforce Pijing 15 times, clear Ganjing 5 times. Pushing of Sihengwen is added for abdominal distension, and manipulation of Neibagua for the presence of sputum.

11. Constipation

Prescription 1: Push Pijing, Dachang and Qijiegu downward, knead Guiwei, rub Duqi, pinch and knead Zusanli. Reducing is applied for a *shi* syndrome and pushing of Liufu is added. For a deficiency syndrome, kneading of Erma and reinforcing Shenjing are added.

Prescription 2: Reinforce Pijing 10 times, clear Dachang 15 times, manipulate the kidneys and spleen 10 times, clear Ganjing 5 times. Pushing of Tianheshui and clearing of Feijing are added in cases of constipation caused by heat.

12. Loss of appetite

Prescription: Push Pijing, manipulate along Neibagua and Banmen, rub Duqi, pinch the spine, knead Pishu, pinch and knead Zusanli, and pinch the spine 3 to 5 times.

13. Abdominal pain (enterospasm)

Prescription: Squeeze and knead Duqi, rub Dujiao, press and knead Pishu, and knead Yiwofeng. Add reinforcing of Pijing and manipulation of Banmen in cases of pain caused by abnormal diet, and add kneading of the spine and pushing of Sanguan in case of pain of the *xu* cold type.

14. Acute convulsions

Prescription: For coma, pinch Renzhong, Ershanmen, Shixuan and Weiling, and manipulate Hegu and Weizhong. For convulsions, manipulate Qianchengshan, Houchengshan, Baichong and Quchi in addition to the above points.

15. Chronic convulsions

Prescription: Manipulate the arm Yangchi 10 times, knead Erma 15 times, reinforce Pijing 10 times, pinch and knead Yujijiao 5 times, and pacify Ganjing 5 times. Add manipulation of Neibagua and Xiaohengwen if the phlegm is excessive, and kneading of Wailaogong is for abdominal pain.

16. Enuresis

Prescription 1: Reinforce Pijing, push Sanguan,

knead Erma and Wailaogong, reinforce Shenjing, pinch and knead Baihui, and knead Dantian and Shenshu.

Prescription 2: For weak constitution, knead Erma 10 times, reinforce Shenjing 15 times, manipulate the spleen and the kidneys 10 times.

For healthy children, clear Pijing and Xiaochang 10 times, push Tianheshui 10 times and clear Ganjing 10 times.

17. Frequent urination

Prescription 1: Reinforce Shenjing and knead Yujijiao, Erma and Dantian.

Prescription 2: Knead Dantian, Shenshu, and push and knead Sanyinjiao.

18. Retention of urine

Prescription: Press and knead Dantian, push Jimen, clear Xiaochang and knead Erma.

19. Prolapsed rectum

Prescription 1: Reinforce Feijing and Pijing, push Dachang, knead Wailaogong, push Sanguan and Qijiegu, and knead Guiwei and Baihui. The clearing method is used for damp heat, but pushing of Qijiegu is removed, and pushing of Sanguan, Liufu and pinching and kneading of Yujijiao are added.

Prescription 2: For damp heat, clear Dachang 10 times, manipulate along Neibagua 10 times, knead Wailaogong 10 times, push Liufu 10 times.

For deficiency of qi, reinforce Dachang 15 times, knead Wailaogong 10 times and Erma.

20. Night sweating

Prescription: Reinforce Pijing and Shenjing, push Tianheshui, clear Banmen, and knead Shending and

Erma.

21. Spontaneous sweating
Prescription: Reinforce Pijing, push Sanguan, and knead the spine and Zusanli.

22. Morbid night crying
Prescription: Divide yin and yang, and knead Yujijiao and Wuzhijie.

For deficiency of the spleen, reinforcing of Pijing, pushing of Sanguan, and kneading of Wailaogong and Yiwofeng are added. For heat in the heart, clearing of Xinjing, Feijing, and pushing of Tianheshui are added. For fright, clearing of Xinjing, Feijing, and Ganjing is added.

23. Parotitis
Prescription 1: Divide yin and yang, push Tianheshui and Liufu, pinch and knead Yujijiao, Yongquan, clear Weijing, press Yaguan, pinch Fengchi and manipulate Jianjing.

Prescription 2: Push Liufu 20 times, clear Weijing 10 times, and push Tianheshui 10 times.

24. Whooping cough
Prescription 1: Clear Feijing and Weijing, pinch and knead Yujijiao and Yiwofeng, manipulate along Neibagua, push Tianzhu, squeeze and pinch Tiantu and push and knead Tanzhong.

Prescription 2: Manipulate along Neibagua 15 times, knead the palmar Xiaohengwen 15 times, clear Weijing 15 times, and push Tianheshui or Liufu 15 times. Kneading of Yujijiao or cupping at Feishu is added during the spasmatic period.

25. Chickenpox
Prescription: For high fever, push Liufu backward

20 times, and clear Weijing 10 times. For cough and irritability, clearing of Ganjing and Feijing is added. For convulsions, kneading of Yujijiao is added.

For low fever, clear Weijing 20 times, push Tianheshui 15 times and clear Feijing 10 times.

26. Infantile infectious hepatitis

Prescription: Clear Ganjing, Feijing and Weijing, and push Tianheshui. In cases of heat, add Liufu; in cases of abdominal diarrhoea and weak constitution, kneading of Erma and pushing of the spleen and kidney are added; in cases of loss of appetite or indigestion, kneading of Banmen is added; in cases of constipation, pushing of the spleen and kidneys is added; in cases of irritability, distension and fullness of the chest, emotional frustration or enlargement of the liver and spleen, manipulation of Neibagua is added.

27. Red and painful eyes

Prescription 1: Push Meigong, manipulate Taiyang, pinch Fengchi, clear Ganjing, push Tianheshui and Liufu, and knead Yujijiao, Shenwen and Yongquan.

Prescription 2: A. Knead Erma 10 times, push Liufu backward 10 times, and pinch and knead Yujijiao 10 times. B. Clear Ganjing and Feijing 10 times, knead Yujijiao 10 times, push Tianheshui 10 times.

28. Sore throat

Prescription 1: Clear Feijing and Weijing, push Tianheshui, pinch Shaoshang, manipulate Hegu, Quchi and Fengchi, and pinch and knead Qiaogong (below the ear to the neck).

Prescription 2: Squeeze Xinjian, manipulate Hegu, pinch Shaoshang or prick the above points with a three-edged needle, and knead the neck.

29. Thrush

Prescription: Reinforce Shenjing, push Tianheshui, knead Zongjin, Yujijiao and the palmar Xiaohengwen, push Xiaohengwen, clear Banmen and Feijing, push Liufu backward, and knead Erma.

30. Delayed closure of the fontanel

Prescription: Reinforce Ganjing, push Sanguan, Pijing and Liufu, and knead Erma. Kneading of Yujijiao and Yiwofeng and pushing of Xiaohengwen are added in cases of shaking head and crying; and pushing of Liufu and clearing of Dachang are added in cases of constipation.

31. Infantile muscular torticollis

Prescription: Knead and pinch the musculus sternocleidomastoideus at the affected area and manipulate Jianjing. Shake the patient's head to radiate the feeling to the affected area.

32. Infantile roundworm-intestinal obstruction

Prescription: Prior to treatment, ask the patient to administer 30 to 50 ml of liquid paraffin or caster oil, then rub the abdominal region rotatively with talcum powder. When the pain is relieved, rotatory kneading is performed. The patient is asked to administer piperazine to drive out the roundworms. If the patient is unable to cooperate due to severe pain, administer or inject intramuscularly an antispastic analgesics like atropine. If abdominal pain is relieved after treatment, but abdominal distension remains, administer a retention enema with soft liquid soap. If the above methods fail, transfer the patient to surgery.

33. Infantile sublaxation of the capitulum radii

Prescription: Put the thumb on the inner side of the

patient's elbow and hold the patient's wrist with the other hand. Keep the palm facing upward and forcefully crook the patient's arm. When the arm is flexed to 90°, a cracking sound is heard, and the joint is repositioned.

34. Infantile health care

Prescription: Reinforce Pijing 200 to 300 times. Rub the abdomen 1 to 3 times, knead the spine 3 to 5 times, and pinch and knead Zusanli 50 to 100 times. Treat 2 to 3 times a week.

VI. Precautions

1. Mediums to be used

In manipulation, apply oil, powder or water to the hands to moisten the skin and strengthen the stimulation. These materials are called tuina mediums or lubricants. Talcum is used in all four seasons, onion and ginger water in winter and spring, and peppermint water or watergreen oil in summer according to the pathological conditions.

2. The reinforcing-reducing method and reinforcing-reducing intensity

The manipulation is divided into reinforcing, reducing and even movement. Reinforcing-reducing is mainly related to the manipulating force and operating speed and direction. Generally, reinforcing is characterized by a light force, slow speed and manipulation along the running direction of the meridian (some specific points have their own particular direction), reducing is just the opposite, and even movement uses a medium force and speed with a back and forth direction.

Reinforcing-reducing intensity is also known as

stimulating intensity, which is closely related to the strength and number of manipulations. Effective reinforcing-reducing intensity is a difficult manipulation problem.

In general, the total time for one tuina manipulation is 10 to 20 minutes, or a little longer. Pushing, rotatory kneading, the rubbing manoeuvre and circular pushing (weak manipulation) are applied to babies at the age of one year.

Manipulate each point 300 times (about 2 minutes). Pinching, pulling, squeezing and spinal kneading (strong stimulation) are applied only 2 to 5 times. The pressing force should be even, gentle, and deep only enough to reach the affected area. The force and number of manipulations should be applied according to the patient's sex, age, pathological conditions and the characteristics of the points.

3. Position

Suitable positions (sitting, supine and recumbent) should be adopted according to the patient's disease, the points to be selected, and the requirements for the operator's manipulations. The positions selected should allow the operator to manipulate freely and the patient to feel comfortable.

4. Tuina sequence

Manipulate in sequence according to the prescriptions to avoid disorders or missing the points. There are three sequences that are used flexibly for different conditions.

1) Manipulate from the upper part of the body to the lower part according to the locations of the points. For example, the points on the head and face are manipulated first, then the points on the upper limbs, chest and abdomen, lumbar region and the lower limbs.

2) The main points should be manipulated before the secondary points.

3) The secondary points are manipulated before the main points.

No matter which method is applied, heavy stimulation by pinching, pulling and squeezing should be performed last to avoid affecting the manipulation and its effects.

The points on the left hand are used for pushing, or are pushed bilaterally. The points on the other regions are generally manipulated bilaterally.

5. The principles of treatment and prescriptions

The basic principles of tuina treatment are the treatment of symptoms and root causes, and warming, invigoration, tonification, reduction, diaphoresis, mediation, resolution and purgation.

The prescriptions consist of manipulations, points and number of times. Main points and secondary points are selected, in which the main points are used to treat the main symptoms, while the secondary points function to strengthen the function of the main points, constrain the function of the main points, and coordinate with the main points to treat some secondary symptoms.

VII. Classification Table for the Commonly Used Tuina Points

Classification	Name of points	Location	Manoeuvre	Manipulating direction	Function	Indications
Points on the Head and Face	Baihui	On the midpoint of the line connecting the apexes of the two auricles	Pinching	Perpendicularly downward	Soothing the nerves, invigorating vital function	Headache, bed-wetting, prolapsed rectum, convulsions
	Xinmen	2 cun anterior to Baihui	Pushing	Perpendicularly	Soothing the nerves and resuscitation	Headache, convulsions, loss of consciousness, irritability, nasal obstruction, rhinorrhea
	Zanzhu	On the medial extremity of the eyebrow	Pushing	Perpendicularly	Dispelling pathogenic wind from the exterior of the body, soothing the nerves and easing the mind	Fever, headache, common cold, lassitude, fright
	Kangong	Directly from the eyebrow to the pupil	Pushing	Parallel	Dispelling pathogenic factors from the exterior of the body, improving eyesight and relieving headache	Fever due to exogeneous affection, convulsions, headache, red and painful eyes

Points on the Head and Face

Point	Location	Manipulating	Method	Indications
Meixin	Between the eyebrows	Pinching	Perpendicularly	Headache, rhinitis, insomnia
Taiyang	In the depression posterior to the eyebrow	Manipulating	Rotatory	Dispelling the pathogenic wind to relieve exogenous symptoms, removing heat and improving eyesight, relieving headache
Shangen	Between the inner canthus of the two eyes	Pinching	Perpendicularly	Resuscitation, improving eyesight and easing the mind
Yannian	On the high bridge of the nose	Pinching	Perpendicularly	Convulsions
Zhuntou	On the tip of the nose	Pinching	Perpendicularly	Resuscitation
Renzhong	Below the nose, a little above the midpoint of the upper lip	Pinching	Perpendicularly	Reducing heat, dispelling wind and resuscitation
Chengjiang	In the depression of the lower lip	Pinching	Perpendicularly	Windstroke, summer heat, loss of consciousness, shock, epilepsy, hysteria, deviated mouth and eyes, toothache, stiff and painful back
Yaguan	1 cun below the ear in the depression of the mandible	Kneading	Rotatory	Dizziness, headache
Erhougaogu	In the depression at the posterior margin of the processus mastoideus	Kneading	Rotatory	Deviated mouth and eyes, toothache

Clenched teeth, deviated mouth and eyes

Dispelling pathogenic wind to relieve symptoms, treating common cold and headache

Headache, convulsions, irritability

Points on the Back

Point	Location	Manipulation	Direction	Function	Indications
Fengchi	In the posterior aspect of the neck, below the occipital bone, in the depression between the upper portion of m. sternocleidomastoideus and m. trapezius	Pinching	Rotatory	Relieving the exogenous symptoms by sweating, dispelling pathogenic wind and cold	Common cold, headache, fever, dizziness; stiff neck and back pain
Xinjian	Between the 2nd and 3rd cervical vertebra	Squeezing and kneading	From both sides or up and down to the centre	Eliminating accumulated heat and clearing the throat	Sore throat, hoarseness
Tianzhu	Along the line from Dazhui upward to the back hairline	Pushing	Perpendicularly	Promoting downward flow of qi, stopping vomiting, dispelling pathogenic wind and cold	Nausea, vomiting, stiff neck, fever, convulsions, sore throat
Dazhui	Between the spinous processes of the 7th cervical vertebra and the 1st thoracic vertebra	Squeezing pinching Kneading	Squeezing and From both sides to the centre Rotatory	Removing exogenous affection, dispelling cold, removing heat from the upper jiao	Common cold, stiff neck, pain of shoulder and back, fever, vomiting
Jizhu	A straight line from the lumbosacrum to Dazhui	Pushing	Perpendicularly	Regulating yin-yang, activating qi and blood, promoting the flow of meridians; nourishing the primary qi	Fever, convulsions, night crying, malnutrition, abdominal diarrhoea, vomiting, abdominal pain, constipation
Feishu	1.5 cun lateral to the lower border of the spinous process of the 3rd and 4th thoracic vertebrae	Kneading	Rotatory	Regulating qi of the lungs, removing deficiency, stopping coughing	Asthma, wheezing, stuffiness of the chest, fever

	Point	Location	Manipulation		Indications
Points on the Back	Pishu	1.5 cun lateral to the lower border of the spinal process of the 11th thoracic vertebra	Kneading	Rotary	Strengthening the spleen and stomach, promoting digestion, removing dampness	Vomiting, abdominal diarrhoea, malnutrition, loss of appetite, chronic convulsions, weak limbs
	Shenshu	1.5 cun lateral to the lower border of the spinal process of the 14th thoracic vertebra	Kneading	Rotary	Nourishing yin, reinforcing yang and kidney qi	Diarrhoea, constipation, pain of lower abdomen, weak lower limbs
	Qijie	A straight line from the coccyx to the 4th lumbar vertebra	Pushing	Up to down or vice versa	Warming yang to stop diarrhoea, dispelling heat and promoting defecation by reducing	Diarrhoea, constipation, prolapsed rectum
	Guiwei	At the tip of the coccyx	Kneading	Rotary	Regulating the function of the stomach and intestines	Warming yang and stopping diarrhoea
	Changqiang	Midway between the tip of the coccyx and the anus	Kneading	Rotary	Regulating the function of the intestines to counter inflammation	Enteritis, hemorrhoids, prolapsed rectum
	Tiantu	In the centre of the suprasternal fossa	Pressing and kneading	Rotary	Removing obstruction from the chest, resolving phlegm and stopping asthma	Cough and asthma, difficult expectoration
Points in the Thoracic and Costal Regions	Shanzhong	On the middle of the sternum, between the nipples	Kneading and separated pushing	Rotary in kneading and pushing in a straight line	Removing obstruction from the chest, stopping cough and resolving phlegm	Cough and asthma, stuffiness of the chest, chest pain
	Rugen	In the intercostal space, one rib below the nipple	Kneading	Rotary	Ditto	Cough and asthma, stuffiness of the chest

Points in the Thoracic and Costal Regions

Rupang	2 cun lateral to the nipples	Kneading	Rotatory	Ditto
Xielei	At the place from below the costal regions to Tianshu	Rubbing	Parallel	Stuffiness of the chest, intercostal pain, asthma, short breath, indigestion, enlargement of the liver and spleen
Zhongwan	On the middle of the abdomen, 4 cun above the umbilicus	Kneading and Rubbing	Rotatory	Resolving phlegm, relieving stuffiness from the chest
Fuyinyang	In the upper abdomen	Separated pushing	Pushing from the xiphoid process	Strengthening the spleen and stomach digestion
Duqi	In the navel	Kneading	Rotatory	Strengthening the spleen and stomach, promoting digestion
Dantian	In the lower abdomen (2-3 cun below the navel)	Kneading or rubbing	Rotatory	Warming up yang to dispell cold, reinforcing qi and blood, strengthening the spleen and stomach
Tianshu	2 cun lateral to the umbilicus	Kneading	Rotatory	Strengthening the kidneys, warming the lower jiao to distinguish turbidity and clarity
Dujiao	2 cun below the umbilicus and 2 cun lateral to the tendinomuscles	Manipulating	Upward	Regulating the function of the large intestine, readjusting circulation of qi and removing food stagnation

				Stuffiness of the chest, cough, wheezing, vomiting
				Abdominal distension, indigestion, vomiting, diarrhoea, loss of appetite, belching
				Abdominal pain and distension, indigestion, vomiting, nausea
				Abdominal distension and pain, indigestion, constipation, gurgling sound, vomiting
				Diarrhoea, abdominal pain, bed-wetting, prolapsed rectum, hernia
				Diarrhoea, constipation, abdominal distension and pain, indigestion
				Abdominal pain, diarrhoea

Points in the Medial Aspect of Upper Limbs and Palm

Point	Location	Manipulation	Direction	Indications
Sanguan	On the radial border of the forearm in a straight line between Yangchi and Quchi	Pushing	Upward	Reinforcing qi, warming up body after illness, weak yang to dispell cold, removing exterior symptoms by sweating, treating xu-cold syndromes
Tianheshui	In the middle of the medial aspect of the forearm in a straight line from Zongjin to Quze	Pushing	Upward and downward	Reducing heat to relieve the exterior symptoms, reducing fire to treat irritability, treating all the heat diseases
Liufu	At the ulna side, on the line from Yangchi to the elbow	Pushing	Downward directly	Reducing heat, cooling blood, detoxication, treating shi-heat diseases
Zongjin	At the midpoint of the wrist crease on the palmar aspect	Kneading	Outward rotation	Reducing heat to remove stagnation
Yujijiao	In the middle of the radial end of the wrist crease of the palmar aspect	Kneading or beating	Rotatory in kneading and beating perpendicularly	Removing the obstruction of orifices, eliminating stasis, stopping convulsions, easing the mind, brightening the vision, reducing heat
Fenyinyang	On both sides of Yujijiao, closing the thumb being Yangchi and closing the little finger being Yinchi	Separated pushing	From Yujijiao to the outside	Balancing yin and yang, regulating the zang-fu organs

Points in the Medial Aspect of Upper Limbs and Palm

Banmen	Below the thumb at the white and red flesh of the radial aspect of the palm	Pushing	Back and forth	Freeing the accumulated qi in the intestines and stomach, reducing stomach heat, stopping vomiting.	Nausea, cholera, vomiting, diarrhoea, milk discharge
Banmen to Hengwen	From the phalangeal joint of the thumb, via the major thenar muscle to the wrist transverse crease	Pushing	To the wrist direction	Strengthening the spleen and stomach	Weakness of spleen yang, diarrhoea
Hengwen to Banmen	From the wrist transverse crease to the major thenar muscle	Pushing	Downward	Relieving stuffiness of the chest, clearing heat in the stomach	Stuffiness of the chest, vomiting
Neilaogong	In the centre of the palm. When the fingers are flexed, the point is between the 2nd and the 3rd metacarpal bones where the index and middle fingers point to	Kneading	Outward rotation	Reducing heat to relieve the exterior symptoms, stopping convulsions	Convulsions due to fright, fever caused by common cold, shi-heat syndromes
Neibagua	At the external circle of the palm	Circular pushing	From inside to outside or vice versa	Promoting the circulation of qi and blood, regulating the zang organs	Cough, diarrhoea
Pijing	At the radial aspect of the thumb from the tip to the root along the white and red skin	Pushing	Straight upward or downward	Strengthening the spleen and stomach by reinforcing, removing food stagnation by reducing	Weakness of the spleen and stomach, loss of appetite, emaciation, listlessness

Points in the Medial Aspect of Upper Limbs and Palm

Name	Location	Manipulation	Direction	Function	Indication
Dachang	At the medial aspect, forming a straight line from the tip of the index finger to the finger web	Pushing	Straight upward or downward	Regulating the function of the intestines by reinforcing and clearing heat and promoting defecation by reducing	Diarrhoea, dysentery, constipation, abdominal pain
Ganjing	On the palmar surface from the tip to the root of the index finger	Pushing	Ditto	Clearing heat from the Liver and Gallbladder Meridians, easing the mind	Convulsion, red eyes, irritability, fright, burning sensation of the palms, soles and heart
Xinjing	On the palmar surface from the tip to the root of the middle finger	Pushing	Straight outward pushing or rotatory reinforcing applied for this point	Reducing heat and fire, no reinforcing	Burning sensation of the palms, soles and heart, convulsions, ulceration of the mouth and tongue, red urine, palpitation
Feijing	On the palmar surface from the tip to the root of the ring finger	Pushing	From the root to the tip of the finger or vice versa	Reinforcing qi of the lungs by reinforcing, reducing shi heat of the lungs by reducing	Common cold, cough, asthma, gurgling sound, constipation
Shenjing	On the palmar aspect of the little finger and a little to the ulna aspect from the tip to the root of the little finger	Pushing	From the tip to the root of the finger or vice versa	Nourishing the kidneys and reinforcing yang by reinforcing, reducing heat in the lower jiao by reducing	Congenital deficiency, weakness after chronic disease, diarrhoea at dawn, bed-wetting, cough and asthma
Xiaochangjing	On the ulnar border of the little finger	Pushing	From the tip to the root of the palm	Reducing heat and promoting urination	Diarrhoea, scanty urine, no urine, high fever, afternoon fever
Xiaohengwen	On the transverse crease of the phalangometacarpal joints of the index, middle, ring and little fingers	Kneading	Rotatory from left to right	Relieving stuffiness of the chest, dissolving phlegm	Ulceration of the mouth and tongue, salivation, cough with excessive sputum, bronchitis, whooping cough, pneumonia and respiratory system disorders

Points in the Medial Aspect of Upper Limbs and Palm

Name	Location	Manipulation		Functions	Indications
Sihengwen	On the transverse crease of the 1st phalangometacarpal joints of the index, middle, ring and little fingers	Pushing or pinching	Perpendicularly from the index finger to the transverse crease of the little finger	Reducing heat, removing irritability, removing blood stagnation	Indigestion, abdominal distension and pain, disharmony of qi and blood, malnutrition, convulsions, asthma, cracked lips.
Shenwen	At the palmar aspect, on the transverse crease of the 2nd phalangometacarpal joint of the little finger	Kneading	Rotatory	Dispelling wind, clearing the vision, removing stagnation	Red eyes, thrush, penetration of heat toxicity
Shending	At the tip of the little finger	Kneading	Rotatory	Astringing the primary qi, stopping perspiration	Spontaneous sweating, night sweating, delayed closure of the fontanel
Yunturushui	From the root of the little finger to the root of the thumb	Yunturushui	Rotatory	Dispelling damp heat in the spleen and stomach, nourishing the kidney water	Diarrhoea, abdominal distension, gurgling sound, indigestion
Yunshuirutu	Ditto	Yunshuirutu	Rotatory	Moisten dryness, removing stagnation	Red and scanty urine, constipation
Shuidiaoyue	Along the border of the little finger from the tip via the root of the palm to the centre (Neilaogong)	Circular pushing	Rotatory	Clearing heat by its cooling property	Heat in the Heart Meridian and heat diseases
Yiwofeng	In the depression in the middle of the wrist transverse crease on the dorsal aspect	Kneading	Rotatory	Relieving the exterior symptoms and dispelling cold	Common cold, nasal obstruction, runny nose, cold pain of the abdomen

Points Along the Lateral Aspect of the Upper Limbs and the Dorsum of the Palm

Wailaogong	In the centre of the dorsum of the hand, opposite Neilaogong	Kneading	Rotatory	Warming up yang to dispel cold, warming the lower jiao	Indigestion, gurgling sound, diarrhoea, dysentery due to cold, abnominal distension, hernia, prolapsed rectum, ascariasis
Weiling	On the dorsum of the hand between the 2nd and 3rd metacarpal bones beside Wailaogong	Pinching and kneading	Perpendicularly for pinching and rotatory for kneading	Resuscitation	Tinnitus, headache, unconsciousness due to acute convulsions
Jingning	On the dorsum of the hand beside Wailaogong, in the depression between the 4th and 5th metacarpal bones	Pinching and kneading	Ditto	Promoting digestion and removing food stagnation	Asthma with excessive sputum, retching, palpable lumps in the abdomen
Erma	On the dorsum of the hand, lateral to Wailaogong, in the depression between the ring and little fingers	Kneading	Rotatory	Nourishing kidney yin and reinforcing yang of the kidney	Dysuria, indigestion, abdominal pain, weak body constitution, prolapsed rectum, bed-wetting, cough and asthma
Tanmen-ruhukou	Along the lateral aspect from the tip of the thumb to the place between the thumb and index finger	Pushing	Straight up and down	Smoothing the flow of qi and harmonizing the blood circulation	Anhidrosis, clenched teeth, sore throat, asthma with excessive sputum
Ershanmen	In the centre of the dorsum of the hand and in the depression between the 3rd and 4th metacarpal bones	Pinching	From both sides of the point to the centre	Relieving the exterior symptoms by diaphoresis, promoting smooth circulation of qi and blood to relax muscles and tendons	Common cold, anhidrosis, asthma, fullness of the chest

Points Along the Lateral Aspect of the Upper Limbs and the Dorsum of the Palm

Point	Location	Manipulation	Direction	Function	Indications
Wuzhijie	On the dorsum of the hand, in the middle of the 5 phalangometacarpal joints	Pinching and kneading	Perpendicularly and rotatory	Resuscitation and stopping convulsions	Convulsions
Laolong	0.1 cun posterior to the nail of the middle finger	Pinching	Perpendicularly	Resuscitation, stopping convulsions, reducing heat and keeping calm	Acute febrile convulsions, especially convulsions with the eyes looking upward, fever, irritability, fright, restlessness, afternoon fever, dull mind, wailing, trance
Duanzheng	On the margin between the red and white skin beside the root of the nail of the middle finger. The one on the radial side is the left Duanzheng and the one at the ulnar side is the right Duanzheng	Pinching	From the both sides to the centre of the point	Ascending for the left point and descending for the right point	Diarrhoea and dysentery by pinching the left point, vomiting and epistaxis by pinching the right point
Shixuan	At the tips of the 10 fingers	Pinching	Perpendicularly	Resuscitation and reducing heat	Acute convulsions, dull mind, morbid night crying
Pangguang	6 cun above Xuehai, corresponding to the area of Jimen	Pulling	Forcefully		Retention of urine

Points of the Lower Limbs

Point	Location	Manipulation	Direction	Function	Indications
Jimen	At the medial aspect of the thigh, forming a straight line from the upper border to the inguinal groove	Pushing	Straight upward	Mild property and promoting diuretic action	Dysuria, retention of urine, watery diarrhoea
Xuehai	At the medial aspect of the thick muscles above the knee	Pressing or pulling	Perpendicularly when pressing and outward when pulling	Removing obstructions from the meridians and stopping spasms	Contracture of the four limbs, weakness of the lower limbs

Points of the Lower Limbs

Name	Location	Manipulation	Direction	Indications
Xiyan	In the depressions of both sides below the patella	Pressing	Perpendicularly	Stopping spasms and easing the mind
Zusanli	3 cun below Waixiyan and 1 cun lateral to the tibia	Kneading and pressing	Rotatory and perpendicularly	Strengthening the spleen and stomach, regulating the flow of qi in the middle jiao
Weizhong	In the centre of the popliteal fossa and in the depression between the two tendons	Pulling	Forcefully	Convulsions, spasms, weakness and atrophy of the lower limbs
Houchengshan	In the depression at the juncture of the musculus gastrocnemius	Pressing, kneading or pushing	Rotatory or straight	Spasm of the gastrocnemius muscles, weakness and atrophy of the lower limbs
Jiexi	On the transverse crease anterior to the ankle, and in the depression between the two tendons	Pinching or kneading	Perpendicularly or rotatory	Convulsions, spasms, constant diarrhoea and vomiting, motor impairment of the ankle joint
Pushen	In the depression inferior to the lateral malleolus	Pulling	From up and down to the centre	Coma, spasm
Yongquan	In the anterior depression of the sole of the foot	Kneading	From outside to inside, rotatory or straight	Fever, vomiting, diarrhoea, burning sensation of the palms, soles and chest
Sanyinjiao	3 cun directly above the tip of the medial malleolus	Pressing, kneading or pushing	Rotatory or straight	Removing obstructions from the meridians, activating the blood circulation, regulating the function of the lower jiao, dispelling damp heat and adjusting water passages

Weakness and atrophy of the lower limbs, convulsions and spasms

Abdominal distension and pain, vomiting, diarrhoea, weakness and atrophy of the lower limbs

Bed-wetting, retention of urine, frequent urination and painful urination

Conducting the fire downward, reducing xu heat

小儿推拿疗法

栾长业 著

单永进 绘图

*

外文出版社出版
(中国北京百万庄路 24 号)
外文印刷厂印刷
中国国际图书贸易总公司
(中国国际书店)发行
北京 399 信箱
1989 年(34 开)第一版
(英)
ISBN 7-119-00641-X/R·13 (外)
00430
14-E-2316P